Acclaim for
The God Prescription

"Avery's passion and dedication are truly phenomenal. He is a calm, kind, and honest presence in the operating theatre. In surgery, he is a true master of what he does. He prepares intensively before surgery and is totally focused. He prays throughout—you can literally watch him talk to God as he works, so he is calmly able to make life and death decisions quickly and efficiently as he works in tiny areas of the brain, where one small move in the wrong direction could mean death or disability. Avery pours this enthusiasm and dedication into this book to help others experience the power of the mind."

—Caroline Leaf, PhD
Communication Pathologist and Cognitive Neuroscientist

"Dr. Jackson's excellent book *The God Prescription* is a must-read. He understands that man is not just a physical or mental being, but a tri-part being: spirit, soul, and body. The failure to be healthy in any of these three areas can produce negative results in all parts of your human system. He shows with empirical evidence that your spiritual beliefs matter. In his book, Dr. Jackson helps the reader to understand that by nourishing your spirit and soul, you can avoid debilitating, costly, and painful illnesses and diseases in your body. I highly recommend this book for everyone."

—Bishop Keith A. Butler
Founding Pastor
Word of Faith International Christian Center Church
Southfield, Michigan

THE GOD PRESCRIPTION

Our Heavenly Father's Plan
for Spiritual, Mental, and Physical Health

Avery M. Jackson III, MD, FAANS

DIGITAL
LEGEND

The God Prescription (2nd Edition)

Permissions & information: info@digitalegend.com

ISBN-13: 978-1-964978-26-0

Published by Digital Legend Press & Publishing, Inc.
Salt Lake City UT

The God Prescription
PO Box 210190
Auburn Hills, Michigan 48321
www.thegodprescription.com
www.thebodyhealthcare.com
draveryjackson.cardiomiraclehealth.com

Contents

Foreword

first spoke with Dr. Avery Jackson when he sent me a lovely
email a few years back in response to my book *Switch on Your
Brain*, in which I talk about the mind–brain connection research I have been doing for the past thirty years and my twen-
ty-one-day brain detox program. I must say, I was thrilled and
honored to get such a wonderful email from such a brilliant
neurosurgeon, who was not only excited about, but also supported my work on how deliberate and intentional thinking
changes the brain (neuroplasticity) and hence our cognitive,
intellectual, social, and emotional health. He especially seemed
excited about the link I showed between science and Scripture
and about how renewing our minds (Rom. 12:2) and bringing
all thoughts into captivity (1 Corin. 5) are essential to mind,
brain, and body health.

Our initial discussions soon grew into a friendship—Avery and
his wonderful family have become family friends. I have had the
honor of interviewing Avery numerous times on my TV show,
"The Dr. Leaf Show," and he is now a part of my Integrated
Mind Network (a team of highly skilled medical professionals
who work together with me to teach and do research on the
mind–brain connection from their various specialties). Avery is
also a regular speaker at my annual conference and is praised by
whoever gets to hear him. I have always loved his enthusiasm for
the mind–brain connection and how he has immersed himself
in all my work—he has been such an encouragement to me! He
is also dedicated to his faith and family and really understands
the link between science and faith.

Avery truly gets it! He sees the importance of how we think, feel, and choose; how this can impact our physical brains and bodies; and how we function in our day-to-day lives. His book is a natural outpouring of his enthusiasm for his love of the brain, his faith, and his own experiences as a child.

Avery's passion and dedication are truly phenomenal. Indeed, one of my favorite things about Avery is watching him work with his patients and watching him do neurosurgery. He has an amazing way of making a patient feel that everything will be all right and that he knows how to help—he instills confidence. He is a calm, kind, and honest presence in the operating theatre. In surgery, he is a true master of what he does. He prepares intensively before surgery and is totally focused. He prays throughout—you can literally watch him talk to God as he works, so he is calmly able to make life and death decisions quickly and efficiently as he works in tiny areas of the brain, where one small move in the wrong direction could mean death or disability. One time, I stood next to Avery for nearly eight hours, watching him successfully remove a tumor from deep inside the brain of one of his patients. I have so much respect for him both as a neurosurgeon and scientist—indeed my respect grew with each passing hour watching him perform intricate neurosurgery like an artist!

Avery pours this enthusiasm and dedication into this book to help others experience the power of the mind. Avery has endorsed my latest three books, and it is a great honor that I am able to write this foreword to his first book!

Caroline Leaf, PhD
Communication Pathologist and Cognitive Neuroscientist

Acknowledgments

I dedicate this book to every child of God who seeks to replace negativity with the transformative love of Jesus Christ, pursuing spiritual, mental, emotional, and physical wellness.

To the God of Abraham, Isaac, and Jacob, my Heavenly Father: You created me with purpose, to share Your boundless love, kindness, and divine will with all humanity. Lord Jesus Christ, my Savior and elder Brother ("and if ye be Christ's then are ye Abraham's seed, and heirs according to the promise," Gal. 3:29, KJV): I thank You for being the embodiment of Truth and the singular Way to salvation. Your redemption, enduring the scourging and wearing the crown of thorns that would have otherwise ensnared my mind and emotions, and shedding Your precious blood, are gifts beyond measure.

To the Holy Spirit: Thank You for Your guidance, politeness, comfort, and power.

I thank God for my wife, Caramarie, who has been a steadfast support throughout this journey of love and dedication. Our family inspires us to work together towards creating a healthier and happier world for all of God's children.

God blessed me with Jeannie Jackson, my mother—an epitome of strength, love, and intelligence. Her guidance from an early age directed me towards God's path for my life. Her unwavering love, especially during challenging times, greatly shaped my journey as a neurosurgeon, where I heal others daily.

I thank God for my sister, Shelley Govan. She embodies a gentle strength and an unwavering faith that shines brightly in every situation. Her presence is a guiding light, showing me how to persevere with grace and positivity through life's challenges.

Dr. Avery M. Jackson Sr., my grandfather, remains a lasting inspiration. His brilliance and boundless energy continue to shape my approach to life and work. I am grateful for the enduring influence of his wisdom and innovation, which drive me forward with a profound sense of purpose and gratitude for the legacy he has instilled in me.

And finally, my heartfelt thanks go out to my esteemed pastors, Bishop Keith A. Butler and Deborah Butler, senior pastors of Word of Faith International Christian Center in Southfield, Michigan. Bishop Butler, founder and president of Keith Butler Ministries (KBM), tirelessly spreads the life-changing message of the Gospel to the farthest corners of the Earth.

Introduction

This book is probably unlike any book you've ever read. It gives you a glimpse into how the mind of a neurosurgeon works when approaching the medical treatment of brain and spine injuries (which have many forms and origins).

As a Christian, I approach medicine from the perspective that God has gifted me with the ability to help heal people. I must, however, rely on His guidance (combined with current evidence-based best practices) to discern the best way to approach every surgery, treatment, and patient discussion.

I am not a pastor or Bible scholar, but I am a true believer in the Holy Trinity—that is, God the Father, Jesus Christ the Son, and the Holy Spirit. That belief informs every aspect of my life and work. I view all of life through the lens of God's Holy Word, the Bible. For that reason, you will see Bible verses sprinkled throughout this book.

The main premise of *The God Prescription* is that God's intricate design of every individual includes three major components:

1. **Spirit:** We are spirit beings because we are made in the image and likeness of God, and He is a spirit.
2. **Soul:** Mind, will, and emotions
3. **Body:** Brain, blood, bones, muscles, etc.

Yet in medical school, we are taught to investigate only the *pathology* of illnesses and diseases—in other words, the structural and functional deviations from the normal that constitute disease or characterize a particular disease. The impact of spiritual and mental/ emotional health on physical health is not typically investigated. In my opinion, this approach addresses only one-third of the human condition.

There is both anecdotal and empirical evidence that demonstrates the significant connection among these three components. Physical disease and illness often appear as the result of mental, emotional, and spiritual issues. As medical practitioners, however, we cannot heal these attributes of the three-part human. Only God can. But He has imparted the *capability* of healing these components, both through self-care and the intervention of trained surgeons and other medical practitioners.

Can you improve your physical health simply by having a positive outlook, attitude, and mind-set? Yes! It's really about your beliefs. What you think about will affect your emotional and physical health. When you feel sick and discouraged, it creates a downward spiral. But if you can turn that negative mind-set around and think positively, you can experience healing. Divorcing His living and life-giving Word, His essence, from the act of "turning the negative mind-set around" will yield less than complete and lasting results.

Blending Science and Scripture to Help Heal Our Bodies

My focus in this book is on the miraculous blending of Scripture with science to heal the human body. I use anatomy and physiology as the basis to help show how God created us for victory and built healing mechanisms into our brains, nervous systems, and endocrine systems from stem cells and genes.

Reading God's Word, the Holy Bible, and focusing on its message of redemption and healing are powerful healing activities. It is important to acknowledge that when Jesus was persecuted, physically tortured, and crucified on the cross, He bore the burden of our sins and all mental and physical diseases.

> But He was wounded for our transgressions, He was crushed for our wickedness [our sin, our injustice, our wrongdoing]; The punishment [required] for our well-being *fell* on Him, And by His stripes (wounds) we are healed (Isa. 53:5, AMP).

As a child of Christ, a born-again believer, you have accepted Jesus Christ into your heart. You acknowledge that He is your Lord and Savior. You acknowledge that He died on the cross for you and then rose from the grave. You are equipped with the most powerful healing capacity there is! Having authority and faith in God's promise and praising Him leads to healing. When we praise God, we forget all the bad things going on in our lives. Our focus changes from thoughts of death to powerful affirmations full of life. The simple act of praising God has healing properties because it changes our focus and splices His Word of life and hope to destroy any destructive thoughts, which then consumes the death-filled thoughts. Once the negative thoughts are consumed, only life is left. Our thoughts are transformed.

> In whom the god of this world hath blinded the minds of them which believe not, lest the light of the glorious

gospel of Christ, who is the image of God, should shine unto them (2 Corin. 4:4, KJV).

For who hath known the mind of the Lord, that he may instruct him? But we have the mind of Christ (1 Corin. 2:16, KJV).

And the peace of God, which passeth all understanding, shall keep your hearts and minds through Christ Jesus (Phil. 4:7, KJV).

It's also important to talk about God out loud to yourself and others. Meditate (which means "to mutter") His words out loud. Being close to God and talking to Him is critical. It will affect your spirit, then your soul, and then your body.

On the science side, having a positive attitude leads to healing. This is true whether you are laughing, stating positive affirmations to yourself, or simply not focusing on the negative reports and words from a credible person, such as a physician. You acknowledge the negative report and then focus on how real God's love is for you based on your past experiences with God, keeping your mind laser-focused on His life-giving words about you and promises intended for you. You will help heal yourself. When God, your doctor, a friend, or a family member tells you, "You are healed, you will be OK, and here are the reasons why," dwell on that encouragement. Don't dwell on the worst-case scenario. Focus on the positive messages until your mind believes them. Once your mind believes healing is possible, your body can respond by healing itself.

Your brain's frontal lobe analyzes the input that enters you through your five senses. The information travels to the hypothalamus, the master gland. Based on input from the frontal lobe, the hypothalamus activates the nervous system, the endocrine system, inflammatory pathways, and the immune system. Worry occurring when the frontal lobe sets the hypothalamus on a trajectory that activates cortisol release and adrenaline and inflammatory pathways, placing a person in survival mode. When doubt, fear, or worry occupy our thoughts for long periods of time, our brains can become stuck in this mode. This leads to emotional, brain- tissue, and body-tissue destruction.

Positive "God" thoughts, however, set the hypothalamus on a different trajectory that signals the rest of the body's systems to create a healing and repairing environment. This, in turn, orchestrates the immune pathways to secrete growth factor such as insulin-like growth factor (IGF).

Isn't that amazing? It is possible because our loving, gracious God created us in His image. And because He loves us. He built in mechanisms to heal our imperfect, earthly bodies, which my pastor calls "Earth suits." As discussed later, the stem cells in our bodies can have a regenerative or reparative function. These same cells, however, can be a destructive force that can act negatively on our own brains and bodies within milliseconds if we allow worry, chronic anger, or self-destructive thoughts to oppress us. We were meant to think positively, both with self-love and love for our neighbors. This love creates the "God environment" within us and around us. God is love. Literally! (1 John 4:8, KJV) God put these stem cells and signals in each of us. He formed us with them when we were two cells old. He knew our bodies would have to endure injury and need a healing process, their original purpose. This demonstrates His love for us!

We Cannot Intellectualize God's Existence

I recognize that not everyone reading this book is a Christian. Some might not even believe God exists. My goal is not to judge anyone but to simply present the path to healing the way I view it as a Christian neurosurgeon. And my goal is not to debate the scientific status of the proposition that "God exists." Some people might not agree with my worldview, but they might agree with empirical evidence and data showing that addressing mental and emotional issues through a spiritual focus can help prevent and even cure physical illnesses.

Medical practitioners and others often debate God's existence based on facts and alleged "proof." The desired proof only takes physical matter into account. This matter, the phenotypical attributes of mankind, accounts for only one-third of our existence. One of the other two-thirds is our spirit, which often goes unrecognized. God is a Spirit that does not exist on a physical plane. We therefore cannot, without distortion, intellectualize His existence or the miracles He performs in our lives every day. Yet that's what we do when we view only one-third of our existence when we think about Him. Instead, we are supposed to utilize all three parts to "see" and interact with Him.

Remember, He made us this way to operate on this earthly plane. We "see" and find God through the medium of faith, spirit to Spirit. God is not bound by time or space. We can find Him only on the plane of faith. Just as we need a diving suit and oxygen tanks to withstand many pounds of pressure under water for long periods of time, so we can exist on the earthly or physical plane only with our interactive five senses and bodies that function well under the force of gravity and atmospheric pressure.

When you think about how each of us is made up of highly complex network of muscles, tissue, organs, cells, and chemical processes, it is hard to argue against God's existence. Each of us began life as two cells and then grew into unique beings, each composed of trillions of cells. Before we can share God's heart and before our spirits can connect with His Holy Spirit, we must acknowledge His existence and trust in faith that He created us in His own image and loves us. Relying only on our limited understanding, we cannot fully comprehend His ways. We can comprehend Him if our hearts—by which I mean one's true self, not the blood-pumping organ—seek Him on the plane of faith, where we can "see" through eyes of trust. In the faith plan of God, we seek and receive wisdom and His peace, which activate our stem cells and physical healing as our spirits become activated and built up by Him and His Words. Proverbs 3:5–8 walks us through our created tri-part nature, providing an illustration of how God intended it to function. The trust is generated by and is an attribute of our souls (mind, will, and emotions). Our hearts are the real us. Our hearts are our core. They are not just a physical blood pump in our chest region. Our navel and bone marrow are some of the parts of our physical bodies. As babies in our mothers' womb, our navels connected the stem-cell-rich placenta to our mothers' bloodstream. Bone marrow is also rich in stem cells, which create and support the immune system when it's nurtured by the appropriate thought environment! Here is the passage from Proverbs:

> Trust in the Lor d with all thine heart; and lean
> not unto thine own understanding. In all thy ways
> acknowledge him, and he shall direct thy paths. Be
> not wise in thine own eyes: fear the Lor d, and depart
> from evil. It shall be health to thy navel, and marrow
> to thy bones (Prov. 3:5–8, KJV).

The infinitely wise God wants us to lean on Him for understanding and daily guidance. Yet we often act like petulant children, insisting on doing things our own way, when we clearly cannot thrive without a relationship with Him. He is the Creator who directed how we were built and how we function. We often take for granted how meticulously and brilliantly He built us. Acknowledging Him should be easy. We can't make a person, not even with the Genome Project. Only God can create the stem cells that He uses to create us.

Like all children, my five-year-old daughter often tries to do things her way. Of course, my wife and I encourage her to try new things and explore her own path in life. But sometimes she's downright stubborn, and her way of doing things doesn't make sense. I tell her, "You are five years old. You don't know what the result of your actions will be. I am ten times older than you. Please understand that I have done all the things you are trying to do, and I am trying to save you trouble and maybe even pain by advising you not to do what you are trying to do."

Likewise, we told my other daughter she couldn't go to her friend's house because she hadn't yet completed her homework. She became distraught, as though this playdate would be the last chance to see her friend. What she didn't know was that I had already rescheduled the playdate with her friend's dad. She didn't have my insight into the situation and therefore didn't have the appropriate perspective on it.

We act the same way with God. We are a fraction of His age, yet we want to do things our way and to tell God, "I don't need You. I know what I'm doing." How arrogant! Who has a greater insight—a 50-year- old or a 50-trillion-year-old (so to speak)?

God loves us. He wants us to acknowledge that there are some aspects of life that are hard to understand. He wants us to "lean not on our own understanding" but instead ask Him to show us how to get from here to there. When you spend time in Scripture and especially pray in the Spirit, in the heavenly language, you will build a personal relationship with Him and be able to discern the direction He wants you to go.

We see the world through the lens of what we know and have experienced. Based on their backgrounds, people react to experiences in different ways.

For example, if someone falls, hitting his head on the corner of a desk, the blood spurting from his head will alarm and upset someone who has never before seen profuse bleeding from such an injury. A neurosurgeon, however, sees bleeding from this area every day and would react to such an accident differently. The surgeon will move quickly to help stop the bleeding and disinfect the wound. The surgeon's heart rate will barely increase, and the stress hormones will return to normal as the situation is stabilized. In contrast, untrained observers of the accident might pass out from panic, even though the situation might not have been catastrophic. Lacking insight into the magnitude of the situation, it traumatizes them instead of spurring them to appropriate action.

Likewise, my experience of being a born-again Christian since the age of twelve causes me to view the world through the lens of God's undying love for us. As a surgeon, I see every day how intricately designed is the highly complex network of muscles, tissue, organs, cells, and chemical processes that structures our bodies. Without a separate act of will, we breathe, think, talk, and walk. It seems miraculous to me, but it's the way God designed us to function. And when we cut ourselves or break a bone, God's brilliant design enables our bodies to heal.

Just raising your arm requires a beautifully intricate orchestration of physical and electrical processes that happen instantaneously in your body and mind. As a neurosurgeon, I see every day how complex and sophisticated God's design is. I therefore cannot separate how I see the world from my understanding that He is our Creator and that He loves us dearly.

If you do not share my beliefs, that is fine. I won't judge you. I do, however, want to share my insight into who God is and how His love works for and in us. I want everyone to know how important awareness of our spirits and the functioning of our souls are to the strength and resilience of our bodies. In fact, we misrepresent God when we hate others because they do not believe what we believe. God loves each one of us and wants us to acknowledge that He exists, that He created us, and that He wants us to lean on Him to guide us through life.

> But without faith it is impossible to please him: for he
> that cometh to God must believe that he is, and that

he is a rewarder of them that diligently seek him (Heb. 11:6, KJV).

Wellness Is a Choice

Research supports the view that by exerting control over our minds and maintaining a positive attitude and mind-set, we are less likely to develop high blood pressure, back pain, auto-immune disorders, and other physical ailments. It is a choice. We must *choose* to claim God's promises, rebuke—that is, express sharp disapproval of—the devil who creates the evil around us, and make decisions that make our spirits, minds, and bodies healthier every day.

When God created Adam and Eve and warned them not to eat the fruit of the tree of the knowledge of good and evil, He knew they would sin and eat from that tree. Why? Because He had equipped them with the gift of choice. But they chose not to follow His guidance. They sinned. That is, they missed the mark, thereby setting the precedent for the future of mankind. Their decision-making process was, as it were, sewn into their offsprings' DNA. Its expression or suppression has depended on the choices of future generations.

Choice is a gift from God. If we want optimal outcomes in life, we must choose to follow God's Word daily and His plan for our lives and well-being.

> For brethren, were [indeed] called to freedom; only [do not let your] freedom be an incentive to your flesh and an opportunity or excuse [for selfishness], but through love you should serve one another. For the whole Law [concerning human relationships] is complied with in

the one precept, You shall love your neighbor as [you do] yourself. [Lev. 19:18.] But if you bite and devour one another [in partisan strife], be careful that you [and your whole fellowship] are not consumed by one another. But I say, walk and live [habitually] in the [Holy] Spirit [responsive to and controlled and guided by the Spirit]; then you will certainly not gratify the cravings and desires of the flesh (of human nature without God).

For the desires of the flesh are opposed to the [Holy] Spirit, and the [desires of the] Spirit are opposed to the flesh (godless human nature); for these are antagonistic to each other [continually withstanding and in conflict with each other], so that you are not free but are prevented from doing what you desire to do. But if you are guided (led) by the [Holy] Spirit, you are not subject to the Law. Now the doings (practices) of the flesh are clear (obvious): they are immorality, impurity, indecency, idolatry, sorcery, enmity, strife, jealousy, anger (ill temper), selfishness, divisions (dissensions), party spirit (factions, sects with peculiar opinions, heresies), envy, drunkenness, carousing, and the like. I warn you beforehand, just as I did previously, that those who do such things shall not inherit the kingdom of God. But the fruit of the [Holy] Spirit [the work which His presence within accomplishes] is love, joy (gladness), peace, patience (an even temper, forbearance), kindness, goodness (benevolence), faithfulness, Gentleness (meekness, humility), self-control (self-restraint, continence).

Against such things there is no law [that can bring a charge]. And those who belong to Christ Jesus (the Messiah) have crucified the flesh (the godless human nature) with its passions and appetites and desires. If we live by the [Holy] Spirit, let us also walk by the Spirit. [If by the Holy Spirit we have our life in God, let us go forward walking in line, our conduct controlled by the Spirit.] Let us not become vainglorious and self-conceited, competitive and challenging and provoking and irritating to one another, envying and being jealous of one another (Gal. 5:13–26, AMPC).

The Hebrew word *shalom* means "wholeness, completeness." Nothing missing, nothing broken. That's an excellent summing up of what we mean by health. God's prescription for having and maintaining good health in all areas of our tri-part existence has everything to do with the choices we make regarding them. We will not get to the root cause of our lack of health without addressing all three.

Physicians often write prescriptions for medications that will cure the disease or at least alleviate the symptoms. This book is my prescription for every man, woman, and child, the gist of which is to acknowledge the profound role of God's guidance, love, and wisdom in our lives. We will never be whole or healthy unless we accept Jesus as our Savior and choose to fill our souls, minds, and hearts with His peace, love, mercy, and grace.

Why I Wrote This Book

God has called me to use neuroscience to spotlight His promises to all of us in the area of healing.

I believe that the God of Abraham, Isaac, and Jacob created the universe and everything in it. His son is Jesus Christ, the Messiah. The Holy Spirit is the third person of the triune Godhead. Each divine person is distinct from the other two, but they are all on the same team.

I believe that God created us in His divine image. As a neurosurgeon, I understand how complex we are. I believe that only God could create such intricate beings composed of sophisticated systems working in tandem to keep our hearts beating, our lungs breathing, and our brains functioning for a century or more.

I wrote this book to help you understand that by nurturing your spirit and soul, you can avoid debilitating, costly, painful, and frustrating illnesses and diseases that manifest as the result of a negative mind- set, emotional issues, and a spiritual void. My goal is to do my part in helping people lead healthier, more fulfilling lives. I believe all the answers to all of life's questions are in the Bible. Go to the Word first, and He will right what's wrong. His Words contain His thoughts—and God's thoughts are powerful. He will strengthen your spirit, which will bring about mental and emotional peace, as well as positive thoughts. And that will lead to physical well-being.

> And let the peace of God rule in your hearts, to the which also ye are called in one body; and be ye thankful (Col. 3:15, KJV).

Only God can truly heal us because healing begins in the soul.

When we recognize that we are children of a loving God who wants only the best for us, we believe in Him and find comfort by communicating with the Lord through prayer and His Word as found in the Bible. That, in turn, heals our minds and emotions. And when our spirit and minds are strong, our bodies are healthy. That is why this book is titled *The God Prescription*. A strong belief in God and a personal relationship with Jesus Christ—the God prescription—leads us to live healthy, happy, productive lives. When we implement God's prescription to address the various afflictions in our spirits and souls (mind, will, and emotions), the body follows and begins to heal.

> The strong spirit of a man sustains him in bodily pain or trouble, but a weak and broken spirit who can raise up or bear? (Prov. 18:14, AMPC).

How My Journey Began

When I was a young boy, my family did not attend church regularly, but I knew that God existed and that He loved us. My maternal grandmother, whom I loved very much, had several strokes. I prayed, "God, please show me how I can help people like her."

When I was eight, God told me, "You are going to be a neurosurgeon." I didn't hear an audible voice. Instead, I heard Him clearly in my spirit, just as we hear from God when we read His Word or receive direction from the Holy Spirit.

"I don't know what a neurosurgeon is," I replied. "But God, I know Your voice, so I'm going to trust You. I will do it."

"I'm going to be a neurosurgeon!" I announced to my teachers, whose reaction was a patronizing nod. Despite that lack of encouragement, however, God had created me to become a neurosurgeon so I could help people. In 1975, I answered that call. That was the year Dr. Herbert Benson discovered "white coat hypertension," the phenomenon of increased blood pressure when one is in the presence of a physician wearing a white coat (see chapter 3). I do not believe the timing of Dr. Benson's discovery (and the ensuing increased understanding of the role of emotions in physical health), just when God was calling me to neurosurgery, was coincidental.

Since then, I have had the urge to pray about this topic, take notes, make observations, and research it. As a Christian, I want to come up with answers and algorithms that can help humanity and address some of the social ills we face. Also, as a physician and as a surgeon, I am fascinated by the physiologic manifestation of illness and disease resulting from a lack of emotional and spiritual well-being.

The training and education took forty years, but now I also have experience in neurosurgery and neuroscience to help me articulate these thoughts and to explain some of what we are seeing today. On March 22, 2015, I was at a church service, and my pastor, Bishop Keith A. Butler, was praying. The Lord told him to tell me, "This is what you're going to do: you will be using your hands to help people who have diseases that are considered incurable, and I will use you to help and bless a lot of people." I will tell you, I take human life very seriously.

God put me on Earth to be a neurosurgeon and to help people. The neurosurgery I do, in and of itself, is a means to an end, not the end itself. It might be a means to our having these conversations and to making a difference in people's lives in ways beyond those that medication or surgery suggests. Understanding the emotional and spiritual basis of disease and illness will enable me to have a greater impact on people, both individually and socially.

My prayer is not only that we will continue to improve our medical management, best practices, and treatment and perform surgeries as needed, but also that we will have a smaller pool of such patients because they will be their own psychological and spiritual surgeons. I hope I can be a catalyst to help open minds and hearts to life-changing thoughts and emotions. This will, in turn, have physiologic ramifications, which will decrease or mitigate the risk of infection, cancer, and autoimmune states. By taking control of your thoughts and your emotions, you can prevent disease and illness. People who understand that they are tri-part beings and acknowledge and support their physical, mental, and spiritual well-being are healthier, overall.

> The *seed* which fell among the thorns, these are the ones who have heard, but as they go on their way they are suffocated with the anxieties and riches and pleasures of this life, and they bring no fruit to maturity (Luke 8:14, AMP).

Improving healthy inter- and intrapersonal relationships is the essence of creating and maintaining the right balance that lets us thrive without experiencing recurrent health issues. This conversation has far-reaching health implications, and it begins and ends with God-given choice!

> I call heaven and earth as witnesses against you today, that I have set before you life and death, the blessing and the curse; therefore, you shall choose life in order that you may live, you and your descendants (Deut. 30:19, AMP).

1

Healing the Tri-Part Human Being Requires a Tri-Part Approach to Treatment

*Is anyone among you sick? He must call for the elders
(spiritual leaders) of the church and they are to pray
over him, anointing him with [a]oil in the name of the
Lord; and the prayer of faith will restore the one who
is sick, and the Lord will raise him up; and if he has
committed sins, he will be forgiven.*
(James 5:14–15, AMP)

Our Heavenly Father has equipped us with the capacity to acquire the necessary skills, knowledge, and tools we need to help heal ourselves and others. However, He wants us to turn to Him for guidance on how to bring about healing.

As a neurosurgeon, I experience the fascinating phenomenon of the tri-part human being every day. When I operate on patients, their lives are in my hands. It is stressful to know that the intricate motions I make with my hands and surgical instruments can help lead to healing and recovery or, if I make the wrong moves, injury or death.

God equipped me with the capacity to acquire knowledge, skills, and education and with the desire to help heal people's bodies. But I cannot rely on my human abilities alone. I rely on the guidance of the Holy Spirit to help me assess life-threatening injuries in seconds and decide on the surgical approach that will minimize complications and result in the desired outcome—the patient's healing and full recovery.

Whether we are operating on brains and spines, raising children, or performing in our jobs, we must recognize that we are tri-part human beings and blend all three components to achieve the best outcome.

First, we must believe and know that God exists and that He created us in His image and equipped us with gifts and abilities, as well as with the ability to choose our own paths. Then we must acknowledge that He loves us and wants the best for us. And then we must listen for His voice and be "clear to hear," as Brother Keith Moore, an amazing teacher of the Word, states. It is critical that we seek His guidance in every decision we make in life.

Reductionist Thinking Doesn't Explain Our Complex Human Makeup

Children suck their thumbs in the womb for comfort. Hmmm. Why would a fetus need comfort? Why doesn't she just float around in her fluid sac until she's born, free from external stimuli? This shows us that a mother's emotional state can affect her fetus. Reductionist thinking will say that we are just cells, and everything happens solely as a result of the environment or solely due to abnormal genes. But that's where the conversation stops.

We are much more complex than that. That's a shortsighted explanation of the results in pathology that we see. Again, when we examine only the pathology of an illness, we are excluding two-thirds of who we are as humans. That approach assumes that the human spirit doesn't exist and that the mind has no bearing on the body.

We have to blend statistical analysis with logic. I am living proof that people can be healed physically by addressing their mental and spiritual lives, as revealed in chapter 2 in my story about recovering from sarcoidosis. I also know of many other people who, despite receiving serious medical diagnoses, chose to think positively and expect healing. As a result, they were healed completely.

Critics and naysayers will say, "They weren't healed because of their God or their thoughts." But the naysayers don't know why those people were healed. Most reductionistic thinkers are brilliant in their fields, but they won't acknowledge that there are certain bits of information that we just have to believe are true, even if unsupported by statistical analysis. We have to believe in some of the science we have that we did not create. We didn't see the original inventors or mathematicians come up with their theories and formulas, yet we believe them. Similarly, we have never seen God, but we need to believe that His Word is true.

Atheists will say that believing in God is hocus pocus, but they believe in the scientific process. They believe in the "null hypothesis," which is kind of a joke. In statistics, a null hypothesis states that there is no significant difference between specified populations and that any observed difference is due to sampling or experimental error. Yet that's the foundation of our science and statistical analysis. We're trying to prove the opposite of what we're disproving. If we can prove the opposite, then we've disproved something; therefore, we've arrived at a major conclusion. Think about how crazy that is. It's not a solid methodology. But we practitioners of science all use null hypotheses in our investigations, in our epidemiology, in our observations, and in the scientific questions we raise and attempt to answer. But it is not foolproof. God's master plan *is* foolproof.

> The spirit of a man sustains him in sickness, but as for a broken spirit, who can bear it? (Prov. 18:14, AMP).

> Do not let your heart be troubled (afraid, cowardly). Believe [confidently] in God *and* trust in Him, [have faith, hold on to it, rely on it, keep going and] believe also in Me (John 14:1, AMP).

God Uses All Things to Work Toward His Purpose

Sometimes when people get sick or injured, they blame God. They assume He doesn't love them or care about them. But God uses all things—even painful experiences and illnesses—to achieve good. He doesn't create these negative experiences or illnesses. We might not see it immediately, but it's all part of His master plan.

> And we know that all things work together for good
> to them that love God, to them who are the called
> according to his purpose (Rom. 8:28, KJV).

God is a loving Father. His intentions and decisions are subject to ours—again, He has equipped us with the ability to make choices. He says we die for a lack of knowledge.

> My people are destroyed for lack of knowledge; be-
> cause you [the priestly nation] have rejected knowl-
> edge, I will also reject you that you shall be no priest
> to Me; seeing you have forgotten the law of your God,
> I will also forget your children (Hos. 4:6, KJV).

But here God is talking not only about intellectual knowledge, but also about knowledge of God, His love for us, and His method of operation. God doesn't create problems; He solves them so that all things work to our good, just as any loving father would do. God imparts divine wisdom to those who are willing to accept it.

Wisdom Comes from Above

As humans, we tend to assess situations based on the physical appearance of systems, actions, or state of being. This is limiting in general, but it is especially so when people make supposi-tions based on their experience or the experience of others and accept it as the final truth.

We are finite beings who can use reasoning based only on our physical senses and information that we analyze in snapshots of time. We often base our interpretation of an event or story on a glimpse of a situation and then jump to a conclusion that is far from the truth. This method *seems* reasonable, but that's because we assume that our "snapshot" of the event is accurate. We conform all other thoughts to that assumed "foundation," which is usually limited to the physical being. It rarely includes the mind or spirit, which is connected to the Holy Spirit, the only One Who sees the whole truth.

Let's say I'm walking in a city. Turning the corner, I observe a horrible scene in progress. A man is grabbing a woman's arm and flinging her to the sidewalk. I immediately assume that the man is the aggressor, the woman his victim. I think, "What a horrible man! I should call the police or intervene."

My reaction, however well-intentioned, was based on the supposition that my interpretation of what I was seeing and feeling was accurate. But I arrived at this conclusion based on my limited physical view of an event in just a sliver of time, filtered through my knowledge of the dynamics of domestic relationships, plus a long-term exposure to the perils of city life.

I could not have the complete truth of the situation unless my heart had been connected with and submitted to the Holy Spirit. Then He could have revealed what really occurred. Maybe the woman slipped and was falling into the path of an oncoming car. The man grabbed her arm, and with all his might, pulled her from certain death, out of the street and toward the sidewalk to safety, just before the car was about to run her over.

In any and all situations, His truth, which is reality, will set us free from the bondage of sin and ultimately death. Everything else is an interpretation of reality through a dimly lit and narrow lens.

God Never Tests Us Harshly

Many people view God as a tyrannical, judgmental, frightening figure who looms high above, looking down on us with disdain and anger and testing our commitment to Him through elaborate, harsh tests. This is far from the truth. Our God is a loving God Who wants only the best for us. He created us in His image!

We can compare God's love for us with our love for our own children. For example, when my five-year-old daughter was learning to read, I knew my wife and I needed to be patient and guide her along, or she'd become frustrated and no longer want to learn. Likewise, she wouldn't learn if we just read to her all the time. We were careful not to "spoon-feed" her because we wanted her to be motivated to develop reading skills at her own pace. This would set a precedent for her to grow and succeed on her own in all life situations, without expecting someone to do things for her.

God does the same with us. He achieves the right balance of teaching us and letting us learn from our own life experiences because He is the ultimate teacher. He uses His resources (His Word, the Bible; Jesus; and the Holy Spirit) to teach us to use all three parts of our being (spirit, soul, and body) to fulfill our desires and needs.

This life is simply an incubator to use physical techniques, including your thoughts, to expose your mind, will, and emotions— that is, your soul—to stimuli that can catalyze growth. God is preparing us for eternal life, just as lifting weights makes us strong internally. Our complexity as tri-part human beings embodies God's design, and He wants us to rely on Him for guidance as we take care of ourselves and others.

Next, I will share with you three stories that demonstrate how God blends my own spiritual, mental (volitional and emotional), and physical abilities to perform life-altering surgeries on my patients.

Patience and Faith Helped Me Remove a Child's Brain Tumor

So how does God equip us to help heal ourselves and others? What does it look like when we apply the concept of the tripart human being to bring about healing?

Our spirits listen to and communicate with God through the Holy Spirit and His written Word. Our souls (mind, will, and emotions) have to be trained or developed in order for us to "hear" the Holy Spirit communicate to us through our spirits. Then we must listen to His voice and respond to the Holy Spirit's leading so that we make choices about how we live that are aligned with His goals for us. This is how the Lord brings about the results He wants for us, for Him, and for other people as we serve them.

We must keep ourselves spiritually in tune with God, mentally alert, and physically fit so that when God calls on us to execute His will, we are ready and able to do so successfully. This requires a combination of patience and faith, and it is up to us to build and strengthen our own patience and faith.

The Lord used the following scenario to build my body and soul. I was assisting in a twenty-four-hour surgery on a six-month old boy. I was in neurosurgery training, learning how to remove brain tumors. My mentor, a senior neurosurgeon, was demonstrating the techniques, and I assisted him in the surgery.

The child had a choroid plexus papilloma—a tumor in the middle of the brain that makes spinal fluid. The middle is very vascular, so this surgery involved a lot of blood. Children have a minimal reserve of blood, so they quickly reach the limit of how much blood loss they can sustain before dying. It was a challenging surgery—not just physically (it took an entire day), but also emotionally.

One Friday morning, we began by opening the child's skull to expose the middle of his brain. We then had to gently move parts of the brain tissue out of the way to create a corridor to the middle of the brain, the location of the choroid plexus tumor, in the *ventricle,* the source of the fluid for the spinal cord.

In this surgery, as in life many times, when you solve one problem, another problem crops up. One series of decisions and choices generates outcomes that then confronts us with new decisions and choices.

As this child's tumor bled a lot, we'd cauterize, or burn, an area for an hour to stop the bleeding so we could remove part of the tumor. This went on for the first seven hours—remove, cauterize, remove, cauterize. We soon were both exhausted. But we didn't want to leave the child alone, nor could we close the skull without risking more bleeding overnight, which would be fatal. We took breaks, sitting in sterilized chairs with our sterile gowns, masks, and hats. We'd allow the work we had done to settle in and some swelling to go down before tackling a different part of the tumor.

The surgery was a success. We removed the tumor, and the child had a full recovery and developed normally.

Patience was the first critical factor. It was critical that we did not rush the surgery and that we remained alert. If we had rushed it because of our own lack of will or intense emotions, or if our minds just went to mush, the child could have died. The second critical factor was that we had enough faith to know that God gave us the skills and tools to do what we needed to do for a successful outcome.

In surgery and in life, the combination of faith and patience is powerful in getting the desired outcome. Patience and faith are required to develop our souls—the mind, will, and emotions—to shore up our mental and physical endurance.

I Had Seconds to Repair an Aneurysm to Prevent a Stroke

Sometimes in life, we have mere seconds to make a critical decision that will have lifelong consequences. This is certainly true in neurosurgery.

I once operated on a fifty-nine-year-old man, a smoker with a family history of aneurysms. An *aneurysm* occurs when part of an artery wall weakens, allowing it to widen abnormally or balloon out. A family member had found him unresponsive at home, and an ambulance rushed him to the hospital. A CT scan revealed a significant amount of bleeding in his brain and an aneurysm in need of repair.

The aneurysm was actively bleeding and 5 centimeters deep. First, I acknowledged the Lord and said, "OK, Lord, I've done this before, but I'm asking for Your guidance and Your peace."

Then I visualized the next steps and stayed alert for the possibility that a complication could arise. I opened the patient's skull with a drill and then opened the covering of the brain. There was some swelling.

I knew I had to stop the bleeding quickly because within seconds, the patient could suffer a stroke and die within minutes. It would be easy to panic, but I was filled with the peace of God. Freaking out would be just as damaging as staying lukewarm and failing to act with urgency. God does not want us to be lukewarm in our faith, either.

> So then because thou art lukewarm, and neither cold nor hot, I will spue thee out of my mouth (Rev. 3:16, KJV).

I could feel my blood pressure rising, which meant cortisol was being released. That enabled me to focus on the next steps. I could feel my pulse in my throat because I knew the heavy bleeding indicated that the patient's aneurysm had re-ruptured. Every adult human body has five liters of blood and can lose one liter within minutes.

If you leave the clips on the arteries too long, the patient will suffer a stroke, the result of a cutoff of blood flow to the brain. Deprived of oxygen, the brain cells begin to die. It's a delicate balance between leaving the clips on long enough so you can see what you need to and removing them before a stroke occurs.

I had to decide—"Am I going to allow my emotions and awareness of unsuccessful surgeries to loop into what could be a horrible scenario in which the patient bleeds out and dies? Or am I going to rely on God to fill me with peace and enable me to fix this problem?" I made the decision to control my emotions. I calmly but quickly placed temporary clips on the blood vessels that supply the main blood vessel to decrease the bleeding so I could see what I was doing. And then I placed a clip on the aneurysm to stop the bleeding.

I left the temporary clips there long enough to give me time to treat the aneurysm and stop the bleeding. The patient's blood pressure stayed stable, and ultimately we were able to close his skull and get him into recovery. He did well after the surgery, but it could have easily gone a different way.

My spirit trusted the Holy Spirit to guide my hands when I couldn't see. And because of the relationship I have with the Holy Spirit, I listened for His voice, the peace of God, during surgery. When we are stressed, our cortisol levels rise, and that can lead to high blood pressure and potentially a stroke. If I had failed to control my emotions, I could easily have suffered a stroke myself as I operated on the patient. Losing a patient is devastating to everyone involved, and knowing that I had only seconds to save the patient's life was incredibly stressful. That's why I turned the situation over to God.

Moving a Fragile Spine the Wrong Way Could Result in Paralysis

Every surgery I perform requires clear, quick thinking and action on my part as a neurosurgeon. I always rely on the Holy Spirit to guide my actions.

I operated on a fifty-year-old-male patient with a crushed spinal cord. He had been complaining about numbness and tingling in his hands, and he had a gait disturbance that caused him to walk unnaturally. An MRI of his back and neck revealed a huge mass that had caused thinning of the spinal cord down to only 20 percent of its original mass.

For the surgery, we placed him on his belly, opened the back of his neck, removed a couple of bones in the back of his spine, and opened the covering of his spine. I exposed the tumor and the spinal cord. His nerves and spinal cord were draped over and under the tumor, which limited my surgical options for removing it.

I wanted to get that tumor out as quickly as possible because once I removed the covering of his spine and the spinal fluid, pressure would begin to build on his spinal cord.

But again, I listened to the Holy Spirit and followed the peace of God within me as I made every decision related to the surgery. That peace was squarely focused on retracting the tumor in one direction and slowly removing large pieces of the tumor with the appropriate instruments.

I was able to remove the entire tumor and saw that his spinal cord in that area was unusually thin. If I were to pull on the tumor the wrong way, I would paralyze his legs and arms.

The surgery was successful, and the patient recovered well. He has full strength and sensation in his arms and legs.

If I had listened to my soul (mind, will, and emotions) only, I would have begun removing pieces of the tumor before doing the proper retraction technique first. If I had acted too quickly, the patient could have become paralyzed. But with the guidance of the Holy Spirit, I was able to control my emotions. I approached the surgery in a way that, at first, didn't seem to be logical, but in the end, was.

Pause to Listen for the Holy Spirit's Guidance

Life is full of urgent scenarios like this. If we follow what the undisciplined soul (mind, will, and emotions) says, we can easily panic and make a costly or even deadly move that leads us down a path of destruction. We must let our human spirits trust the Holy Spirit to take over and guide our actions.

> The Lor d also will be a refuge *and* a stronghold for the oppressed, a refuge in times of trouble; and those who know Your name [who have experienced Your precious mercy] will put their confident trust in You, for You, O Lor d, have not abandoned those who seek You (Ps. 9:9–10, AMP).

When we are faced with a stressful situation, the "fight or flight syndrome" compels us to act quickly without first checking in with our intuition (the Holy Spirit speaking to our true self, our inner person.). When faced with adversity, we often act out of panic in an attempt to fight or flee the source of the adversity.

But again, our Heavenly Father equipped us with the mechanism to make choices. And the better choice is to make a quality decision about how to approach a problem while relying on the Holy Spirit for guidance, wisdom, and discernment.

Let's say you get into an argument with a spouse or coworker, and it leads to a physical or emotional fight. Your soul (mind, will, and emotions) might be telling you, "You need to tell him off because he is wrong." Or maybe you encounter a road-rage situation in traffic, and you feel compelled to act aggressively. Resist that urge! Instead, rely on your relationship with the Lord, and remember that He wants us to be kind one to another.

> And be ye kind one to another, tenderhearted, forgiving one another, even as God for Christ's sake hath forgiven you (Eph. 4:32, KJV).

Life and death are in the power of the tongue, and if you can control your tongue, you control your entire body. Also, by controlling your tongue, you can save the relationship and prevent yourself and others from being harmed. You are controlling your emotions because of your relationship with your Heavenly Father, who cares for you. Again, it is a *choice*. Making a choice deliberately to turn your stressful situations over to your Heavenly Father can make a world of difference in terms of the outcome. Many times, it's a matter of life and death.

We must know who we are— that we are children of God. If we don't know who we are, we won't walk in the authority to be able to make wise choices. What helps ground me is the fact that I know who I am in Christ. I know I can do all things through Christ, which means I can control my emotions, even if being angry is warranted. Without God, I would not be able to do that.

> I can do all things through Christ which strengtheneth me (Phil. 4:13, KJV).

The God Prescription: Strategies to Help Heal Illness by Focusing on the Tri-Part Human Being

1. Acknowledge that our complexity is part of God's design and that He wants us to lean on Him for divine guidance as we allow Him to heal ourselves and others.

2. Understand that God has all things working together for our good and His purpose. When you or someone you care about becomes sick, refrain from blaming God or assuming He doesn't care. Pray for understanding, comfort, and guidance.

3. Recognize that God's vision is truth. Connect your heart with the Holy Spirit, out of a motivation and posture of love, submission, and connectedness through a continuous (not episodic) relationship with Jesus Christ.

2

Focusing on the Spirit-Mind-Body Connection Helps Heal Illness

M any illnesses that lead to premature death are preventable. Nearly 75 percent of all deaths in the United States are attributed to just ten causes, with the top three accounting for more than half of all deaths.

Here are the top ten leading causes of death in the United States, based on 2016 data:[1]

1. Heart disease
2. Cancer
3. Chronic lower respiratory disease
4. Accidents
5. Stroke
6. Alzheimer's disease
7. Diabetes

---

1. Hannah Nichols, "The Top 10 Leading Causes of Death in the United States," *Medical News Today*, February 23, 2017, https:// www.medicalnewstoday.com/ articles/282929.php.

8. Influenza and pneumonia

9. Kidney disease

10. Suicide

Every day, I work with patients whose spiritual, mental, emotional issues manifest in their bodies as illness.

Marie's Chronic Infections Originated in Depression

One of my patients, Marie, is eighty years old. She has a history of severe depression that has led to a breakdown of her immune system, leading to multiple infections. I have operated on her lower back, and other physicians have performed surgery on her as well.

Marie usually ends up with multiple, recurrent infections after surgery due to her poorly functioning immune system, secondary to depression. In fact, some surgeons in my area will not operate on her because they know she will develop an infection.

Why does this happen? Marie's emotions and life decisions create a chronic environment of stress, doubt, and worry, stemming from depression. The chronic cortisol release (fight-or-flight state) and misactivation of her immune pathways lead to a poorly functioning immune system.

There is significant support in the scientific literature confirming that depression leads to increased risk of infection.

We can overcome this common scenario. Satan, our enemy, places pressures, fears, and cares on our hearts and minds daily to separate us from God. But we don't have to accept or keep them! We can cast them off with the Holy Spirit's guidance.

We cannot receive divine peace to nullify those fears without Jesus and without the Holy Spirit's guidance from the Heavenly Father.

In other words, you will be ineffective in fending off the enemy without acknowledging the Lord's guidance internally. You have the peace of God in any situation. His joy is in you and on you, and others can readily see it in you. This is especially true when those individuals who don't know Jesus see your calm, confident attitude and wisdom in difficult situations that would create cynicism and despair in an undisciplined soul.

When the peace of God fills your spirit and soul, then you will handle adversity with wisdom and prudence, and you will refrain from blaming others or lashing out at them when you are hurting.

By this everyone will know that you are My disciples, if you have love *and* unselfish concern for one another (John 13:35, AMP).

You will have so much peace internally that it spills outside of you for others to see and enjoy. You will encourage others to seek God's peace by the behavior you model.

What About Environmental and Genetic Factors?

Emotional stress is not the sole cause of illness. There can be environmental etiologies (or causal explanations). For example, people who live by power lines are more likely to develop lymphoma.

Here is an example of an environmental cause of disease. The little town of Mossville, Louisiana, is near an oil refinery, several petrochemical plants, and one of the country's largest concentrations of manufacturers of vinyl chloride, a main ingredient in polyvinyl chloride, the plastic known as PVC. These facilities emit millions of pounds of toxins into the air, water, and soil each year.[2]

In 1998, a group of residents who organized under the name MEAN—Mossville Environmental Action Now—with the help of Greenpeace, fought hard to convince a federal agency within the Centers for Disease Control and Prevention to conduct toxicological testing. The Agency for Toxic Substances and Disease Registry, ATSDR, drew the blood of twenty-eight Mossville inhabitants. The community's toxicology results were staggering: the average dioxin level among the Mossville cohort was triple that of the general US population. The median level exceeded the country's 95th percentile. Many people in the hamlet, with a population of about five hundred, experienced serious chronic illnesses.[3]

In humans, dioxins can cause cancer, damage the reproductive system, impair the immune system, and disrupt normal hormone functions, which can lead to diseases such as diabetes. Dioxins are resistant to metabolism, so they can build up in the body, wreaking havoc for years. Despite the findings, and despite a respected environmental medicine specialist calling

2. Heather Rogers, "Erasing Mossville: How Pollution Killed a Louisiana Town," *The Intercept*, November 4, 2015, https://theintercept.com/2015/11/04/erasing-mossvillehow-pollution-killed-a-louisiana-town/.
3. Ibid

for action in Mossville, the ATSDR downplayed the findings and refused to take action.

Apparently, no one wanted to take responsibility for the human suffering caused by the manufacturing plants.[4]

We know that smoking and a poor diet can damage our bodies. A diet of unhealthy foods can keep the immune system and stem cells busy for years until both systems become overwhelmed and we lose their protective mechanisms altogether.

Many people think there is a genetic component to some illnesses. I am leery about the genetic arguments because in cases in which a gene is found to cause an abnormality, why did that gene express? Or why *didn't* a gene express? It could be that an internal agent created a gene expression. We know certain genes can express, thereby creating many illnesses, but what causes the genes to express abnormally? I believe emotional distress, physical ingestion, or exposure can be the cause in many cases. More research needs to be conducted, and we need the appropriate collaborative effort among various groups.

If a baby is diagnosed with a disease, we don't know where the disease originated. What happened while the child was in the mother's womb? The baby was not exposed to physical elements in the environment before she was born. But she was exposed to her mother's immune system, directly or indirectly. And she was exposed to her mother's blood, the baby's source of nutrition. What was the mother's emotional state before she conceived the baby, when she conceived, and while the fetus was developing? How do the mother's emotions affect the child?

---

4. Ibid

Let's examine some illnesses and conditions that cause us, as individuals and societies, immense pain and suffering. Please note that every illness and condition known to mankind can be healed by addressing the tri-part human being: spirit, soul (mind, will, and emotion), and physical body.

Suicide

Suicide has increased at an alarming rate over the past two decades. Suicide rates increased more than 30 percent in half of all states since 1999, according to a June 2018 report from the Centers for Disease Control (CDC). Nearly 45,000 lives were lost to suicide in 2016, and more than half of the people who died by suicide did not have a known mental health condition.[5]

Every decision we make—and we make many every day—affects our relationships. Nothing of significance occurs outside the context of relationships! This includes our relationships with others; with ourselves as tri-part beings; and with God the Father, the Holy Spirit, and Jesus Christ, our Lord and Savior.

If your spirit is strong, then you are subject to the positive state of being and can live a carefree life, being satisfied with all those relationships in your life. And that will have a positive effect on your spiritual, emotional/mental, and physical health.

Successful, strong relationships require that we treat one another kindly and love one another unselfishly.

---

5. "Suicide Rising Across the US," Centers for Disease Control, June 2018, https://www.cdc.gov/vitalsigns/pdf/vs-0618-suicide-H.pdf.

So, as God's own chosen people, who are holy [set apart, sanctified for His purpose] and well-beloved [by God Himself], put on a heart of compassion, kindness, humility, gentleness, and patience [which has the power to endure whatever injustice or unpleasantness comes, with good temper]; bearing graciously with one another, and willingly forgiving each other if one has a cause for complaint against another; just as the Lord has forgiven you, so should you forgive. Beyond all these things put on and wrap yourselves in [unselfish] love, which is the perfect bond of unity [for everything is bound together in agreement when each one seeks the best for others] (Col. 3:12–14, AMP).

In fact, relationships with other people and with Jesus Christ are key in preventing suicide.

The CDC confirms the importance of "connectedness" in preventing suicide. A CDC report defines *connectedness* as "the degree to which an individual or group is socially close, interrelated, or shares resources with other individuals or groups." The report says, "Strong, positive relationships with others can be protective and prevent against suicidal thoughts and behaviors. Connectedness between individuals can lead to increased frequency of social contact, lowered levels of social isolation or loneliness, and an increased number of positive relationships."[6]

God loves us and wants us to build ourselves up for Him and for one another. People need to connect with one another and

---

6. "Preventing Suicide Through Connectedness," Centers for Disease Control, https://www.cdc.gov/ViolencePrevention/pdf/ASAP_Suicide_Issue3-a.pdf.

know they are loved. We tend to hold a lot of issues against each other. We can't do that going forward.

> Be ye therefore followers of God, as dear children; And walk in love, as Christ also hath loved us, and hath given himself for us an offering and a sacrifice to God for a sweet smelling savour (Eph. 5:1–2, KJV).

Whether it's suicide or any other condition or illness that plagues our society today, we can find the root cause of that problem in the fact that practitioners tend to focus only on the *physical* symptoms of an illness, or its pathology. The *root causes* of illnesses and the underlying emotional and spiritual well-being of patients are often ignored. Also ignored is a focus on the powerful healing attributes of a positive attitude, prayer, and the hope we can derive from Scripture and a close walk with our Creator.

> The effectual fervent prayer of a righteous man availeth much (James 5:16, KJV).

Stress and Depression

Stress and depression are rampant in our society. These conditions have been associated with worse outcomes in immune-related disorders, including cancer and infectious diseases. This suggests that the effects of these conditions on the immune system are clinically relevant to disease expression.

There is strong evidence that depression involves alterations in multiple aspects of immunity that may contribute to the development or exacerbation of several medical disorders and may play a role in the pathophysiology of depressive symptoms. Accordingly, aggressive management of depressive disorders in medically ill populations or individuals at risk for disease may improve disease outcome or prevent disease development.[7]

We can disrupt the hold that depression can have on us when we focus on God's supreme love for us.

> And the peace of God [that peace which reassures the heart, that peace] which transcends all understanding, [that peace which] stands guard over your hearts and your minds in Christ Jesus [is yours]. Finally, believers, whatever is true, whatever is honorable and worthy of respect, whatever is right and confirmed by God's word, whatever is pure and wholesome, whatever is lovely and brings peace, whatever is admirable and of good repute; if there is any excellence, if there is anything worthy of praise, think continually on these things [center your mind on them, and implant them in your heart] (Phil. 4:7–8. AMP).

When we are under stress, we must focus on God's love for us so that we can address issues in our lives head-on. That will help us break the chronic cycle of stress and relieve us of the heightened physical manifestation of the fight-or-flight syndrome. By consciously controlling our stress, we are better able to live healthy lives in our spirits, minds, and bodies.

---

7. C. L. Raison, et al., "The Neuroimmunology of Stress and Depression," *Seminars in Clinical Neuropsychiatry 6*, no. 4 (October 2001), 277–94.

Psychoneuroimmunology: The Connection Between Stress and Illness

Psychoneuroimmunology (PNI) is a relatively new field of study of the way the central nervous system (CNS) and the immune system interact. The nerves in the brain and spinal cord make up the CNS, while the immune system is made up of organs and cells that defend the body against infection.

Both systems produce small molecules and proteins that act as messengers between the two systems. In your CNS, these messengers include hormones and neurotransmitters. The immune system uses proteins called cytokines to communicate with the CNS. Research has shown that stressful experiences during childhood can increase the immune system's release of cytokines, which is associated with an increased risk of mental illness in adulthood. A 2011 review exploring the link between stress and the immune system found that stress may play a role in conditions that affect the immune system, such as cancer, HIV, and inflammatory bowel disease.[8]

The onset of at least 50 percent of autoimmune disorders has been attributed to "unknown trigger factors." Physical and psychological stress has been implicated in the development of autoimmune disease, and numerous animal and human studies have demonstrated the effect of various stressors on immune function.[9]

---

8. "Understanding Psychoneuroimmunology," Healthline newsletter, https://www.healthline.com/health/psychoneuroimmunology.

9. L. Stojanovich and D. Marisavljevich, "Stress as a Trigger of Autoimmune Disease," *Autoimmunity Reviews 7*, no. 3 (January 2008): 209–13.

Stress Can Lead to Autoimmune Disease

Studies have shown that up to 80 percent of patients report uncommon emotional stress before disease onset. Not only does stress cause disease; the disease causes significant stress in patients, creating a vicious cycle.

Many physicians and researchers believe that stress-triggered neuroendocrine hormones lead to immune dysregulation, which can result in autoimmune disease because of altered or amplified cytokine production. *Cytokines* are substances, such as interferon, interleukin, and growth factors, that are secreted by certain cells of the immune system and influence other cells.

I believe the treatment of autoimmune disease should include stress management (which, of course, includes having the joy of the Lord as your strength) and behavioral intervention to prevent stress-related immune imbalance.

> Then [Ezra] told them, Go your way, eat the fat, drink the sweet drink, and send portions to him for whom nothing is prepared; for this day is holy to our Lord. And be not grieved and depressed, for the joy of the Lord is your strength and stronghold (Neh. 8:10, AMP).

Esther Sternberg, MD, a rheumatologist and now a Senior Investigator in Neuroscience at the NIH, has reflected on the fact that research over the years has led to an improved understanding of the mind–body connection.

We now have improved methods to visualize communication between the central nervous system and the immune and endocrine systems. Dr. Sternberg describes this evolution:

An obstacle to acceptance in the 1980s was that researchers lacked the tools, such as recombinant cytokines, to understand the connection without the possibility of contamination. Without recombinant proteins, it was difficult to show incontrovertibly that immune molecules could change the brain and vice versa. By the mid-1990s, the field had accumulated a critical mass of papers, and it started becoming acceptable to associate with psychologists...By then, enough good research had hit the radar screen so that even skeptics began to take note. From where I sit, there's been a sea change in acceptance of this field.[10]

Two additional researchers who have contributed much to understanding how stress affects the immune system are immunologist Ronald Glaser, PhD, and psychologist Janice Kiecolt-Glaser, PhD, from Ohio State University in Columbus. While studying the Epstein–Barr virus, Dr. Glaser observed that stress seemed to affect its latency. The two researchers first studied how stress in medical students makes them susceptible to infection, and later, how short-term stress negatively affects wound healing by disrupting the production of pro-inflammatory cytokines. More recently, they showed that stress increases the pro-inflammatory response in caretakers of Alzheimer's patients. Dr. Glaser writes, "An increase of pro-inflammatory cytokines with aging is normal, but these chronically stressed caretakers had a six-fold increase in these cytokines over the controls."[11]

---

10. Vicki Brower, "Mind–Body Research Moves Towards the Mainstream."

11. Ibid

The research of Bruce McEwen, PhD, head of the neuroendocrinology lab at The Rockefeller University in New York City, has also shown that stress hormones have dual effects on the brain. They are protective in the short term but damaging in the long term because they impair nerve cells in certain areas of the brain. He developed the concept of "allostatic load"— damaging changes that can accumulate in response to stress because of the adverse effects of overexposure to neural, endocrine, and immune stress mediators on various organ systems.[12]

Stress Caused by Sin and Unforgiveness Can Lead to Damaging Emotions

Sometimes stress and depression result from sin we haven't repented of. By acknowledging our shortcomings and sins, confessing them to God, and asking for forgiveness, the weight of those sins is released from us. Christ died on the cross for our sins. They have already been paid for!

Unforgiveness also can lead to stress and depression. One of the greatest challenges of being human is to forgive people who have wronged us. For some reason, we want to hold on to the negative emotions associated with feeling slighted or hurt. When we refuse to forgive others, we are clinging to toxic emotions that can cause damage to our spiritual, mental, and physical health over time.

Plus, God commands us to forgive others, or He cannot forgive us.

> But if you do not forgive others [nurturing your hurt
> and anger with the result that it interferes with your

12. Ibid

relationship with God], then your Father will not forgive your trespasses

(Matt. 6:15, AMP).

When I was about nine years old, my "mortal enemy" in elementary school was a kid named Kevin. I was a dork, and he was a bully.

One day, Kevin and I were sitting across from each other on a long, white picnic-bench lunch table. The bench was loaded with fifteen kids on each side of the table in the school cafeteria. We were all eating lunch and talking.

Suddenly, the background noise of the three hundred children in the cafeteria melted away. The Holy Spirit filled me with peace, love, and forgiveness—and then alertness. I saw Kevin choking on a stick of candy. He couldn't speak, and he grabbed his throat (the universal sign of "I'm choking"). The next ten seconds seemed to go into slow motion. I ran to the other side of the table, stood behind Kevin, and performed the Heimlich maneuver, which I had recently seen someone do on TV. The candy shot out of Kevin's mouth. He took a deep breath and looked at me, his face beaming gratitude and humility. After that moment, we became best friends.

Pray for those who spitefully use you, disrespect you, and harm you. In fact, the more a person has hurt you, the more important it is for you to forgive him or her. The worse the person's transgression against you, the more difficult it is, but the more peace you will experience by doing so. You'll also avoid inflammatory responses that can be destructive to your body and brain.

Follow Jesus's example. As He was nailed to the cross, suffering a horrific death so that we might live and be forgiven of our sins, He forgave the ones who were crucifying Him. If He can do that, certainly we can forgive those who act with vengeance toward us.

> When they came to the place called The Skull, there they crucified Him and the criminals, one on the right and one on the left. And Jesus was saying, 'Father, forgive them; for they do not know what they are doing' (Luke 23:33–34, AMP).

Sarcoidosis

I know from personal experience that God can heal our bodies by first healing our spirits because I was healed of sarcoidosis.

> The strong spirit of a man sustains him in bodily pain or trouble, but a weak and broken spirit who can raise up or bear? (Prov. 18:14, AMPC).

When I began medical school in 1990, I was diagnosed with sarcoidosis, an inflammatory disease. My parotid glands (salivary glands deep in my cheeks) began to swell. I was under extreme stress but didn't know if this disease was caused by stress or the old apartment building I was living in. I am confident that stress played a major role by causing my immune system to overreact.

I was treated with steroids and began to focus on stress- management initiatives, including time in prayer with my Heavenly Father, Tai Chi, rest, and as much time with family as I could muster.

This is an example of a disease process borne from a weak spirit, leading to a weak mind, in response to a massive emotional stressor (medical school), resulting in the autoimmune disorder called sarcoidosis.

This disease process would present itself during times of extreme spiritual, emotional, and physical stress. I was able to destroy this physical manifestation in response to duress by building up my spirit man, first and foremost by relying on God's Word and promises for my life. This brought me extreme peace.

> And the peace of God [that peace which reassures the heart, that peace] which transcends all understanding, [that peace which] stands guard over your hearts and your minds in Christ Jesus [is yours] (Phil. 4:7, AMP).

I studied God's promises and then prayed in my heavenly language, which filled and strengthened my "inner" man, or spirit man. This gave me power to control my soul (mind, will, and emotions). My perspective regarding the situation changed, even though my circumstance didn't change. My strong inner man then controlled my soul (mind, will, and emotions), which then brought my body under subjection. As a result, I thwarted my physical body's hyperactive autoimmune response.

Now I build up my strength *before* stress comes my way so that when it does, I'm prepared. I prepare by spending quality time with God and God's Word. I focus on how much He loves me and how wonderfully and fearfully He made me. I pray in my heavenly language, which replenishes my inner strength. Then I exercise my body and do good for someone until I experience slight discomfort (reflecting the law of seed, time, and harvest).

These purposeful, positive acts engage all three parts of my being. I have a conversation with God and then trust Him and thank Him. I know that He will take care of the situation. The healing mechanisms and auto-regulatory processes calm my immune system. This creates micro adjustments that bring healing through the genomic blueprint that the Lord created in my body before I was two cells old.

> Before I formed you in the womb I knew you [and approved of you as My chosen instrument], And before you were born I consecrated you [to Myself as My own]; I have appointed you as a prophet to the nations (Jer. 1:5, AMP).

A recent scientific article describes sarcoidosis as "a multisystem disease process of unknown etiology whose pathogenesis involves formation of an inflammatory lesion known as a granuloma. Histologically, noncaseating granulomas are prominent in biopsies from lymph nodes or affected organs. The lungs are affected most frequently, but the eyes, nervous system, heart, kidneys, bones, and joints also may be affected."[13]

Most patients with sarcoidosis have no symptoms; the disease often is detected with a routine chest radiograph. Symptoms, if present, include cough, shortness of breath, and arthritis. Involvement of the central nervous system, or neurosarcoidosis, occurs in 5 to 15 percent of cases of sarcoidosis.[14]

---

13. Gabriel Bucurescu, MD, and Amer Suleman, MD, "Neurosarcoidosis," Medscape, December 7, 2017, https://emedicine.medscape.com/article/1147324-overview.

14. Ibid

Debate continues as to whether sarcoidosis results from a dysfunctional immune system or a secondary response to environmental antigens. Sarcoid granulomas may be seen in solid organs such as the liver, kidney, and spleen.

The causes of sarcoidosis are not clear. Present evidence suggests that active sarcoidosis results from an exaggerated cellular immune response to either foreign or self-antigens. T-helper lymphocytes proliferate, resulting in an exaggerated response.

Three hypotheses have been proposed to explain the mechanism, as follows:

1. A persistent antigen (either foreign or self) triggers the T-helper cell response.

2. Response of the suppressor arm of the immune response is inadequate and cannot prevent T-helper cells from shutting down.

3. A possible inherited or acquired (genetic) difference in response genes leads to the exaggerated response.

Many patients with this disease have a slowly progressive chronic course with intermittent exacerbations. Sometimes brain-stem involvement can be life-threatening. Cases of sudden death have been attributed to cardiac sarcoidosis and hypothalamic infiltration. There is no known cure for sarcoidosis, but physicians often treat the symptoms with various medications that suppress the immune system.

So, although science cannot explain what causes or cures sarcoidosis, I know from experience that I can eradicate it by maintaining a positive attitude, a by-product born of fullness of His Words in my heart until joy overflows through my faith and relationship with Jesus Christ.

Opioid Addiction

Opioid abuse has become an epidemic in the United States, ruining lives, marriages, and careers. Individuals with Medicare Part D are among some of the most affected. As of 2016, one in three Medicare Part D beneficiaries had received at least one prescription for opioids, and one in ten received prescriptions for regularly scheduled opioids.

Due to this increased health safety concern, public health programs such as the Centers for Medicare and Medicaid Services (CMS) and the Centers for Disease Control (CDC) have launched an extensive investigation to find a solution to this epidemic. CMS has started numerous initiatives to investigate patients and prescribers affected by this epidemic. For that reason, the CDC has issued new guidelines for prescribers to follow to reduce opioid abuse, especially in patients on Medicare Part D.[15]

Deaths from drug overdoses in the United States increased 21 percent in 2016. Government statistics released in December 2017 revealed that there were about 63,600 drug-related deaths in 2016, up from about 52,000 in 2015. For the first time, the powerful painkiller fentanyl and its close opioid cousins

---

15. Kelsey Boyle, Jon Heald, and Janis Coffin, "Opioid Abuse: Understand Guidelines to Protect Patients and Your Practice," *Medical Economics*, May 30, 2018, http://www. medicaleconomics. com/business/opioid-abuse-understand-guidelines-protect-patients-and-your-practice.

played a bigger role in the deaths than any other legal or illegal drug, surpassing prescription pain pills and heroin. In fact, two-thirds of the 2016 drug deaths—about 42,000—involved opioids, a category that includes heroin, methadone, prescription pain pills like OxyContin, and fentanyl. Fatal overdoses that involved fentanyl and fentanyl-like drugs doubled in one year, to more than 19,000, mostly from illegally made pills or powder, which is often mixed with heroin or other drugs. Heroin was linked to 15,500 deaths and prescription painkillers to 14,500 deaths.[16]

Why is this happening, and what is the solution?

The answer lies in the complex field of neuropsychic immunology, which we previously noted as psychoneuroimmunology (PNI).It's the study of the interaction between psychological processes and the nervous and immune systems of the human body. PNI combines many disciplines, including behavioral medicine, endocrinology, genetics, immunology, infectious diseases, molecular biology, neuroscience, pharmacology, physiology, psychiatry, psychology, and rheumatology.

When a twenty-three-year-old goes to the doctor for his back pain, with no apparent cause, that condition might manifest because of a trauma he has carried with him for most of his life. The prefrontal cortex of the brain doesn't fully develop until people are in their mid- to late twenties. So a young person won't fully process childhood experiences until then.

------

16. "Soaring Opioid Drug Deaths Cause US Life Expectancy to Drop for Second Year," CBS News, December 21, 2017, https://www.cbsnews.com/news/opioid-fentanyl- overdose-deaths-us-life-expectancy-drops-for-second-year/.

Society will look for a physical source of the back pain, and a doctor might prescribe a narcotic or an opioid to relieve the pain, when in fact, the pain began to manifest years earlier as emotional trauma. This means the back pain has an emotional, causal backstory. The patient might get some relief from the narcotic, but it's more of a placebo effect because someone cared enough to do something for him that he considers substantial. The placebo effect provides temporary relief from the back pain, but when the pain returns, he goes to the doctor again. The doctor says, "Well, the narcotic gave you relief before, so I'll give you more narcotics."

This is one of the many scenarios contributing to our opioid epidemic. Michigan, where I work, is ranked eighth among all states for the most deaths due to opioid abuse. More opioid prescriptions are written each year in this state than the number of people who live in it. This is a downward spiral of destruction to individuals and society. We must address this monumental problem at its origin.

How Physicians Can Reduce Opioid Addiction

A huge responsibility for the opioid crisis falls on the shoulders of the physicians who prescribe these powerful drugs. I urge my fellow physicians to follow these guidelines in an effort to control the opioid crisis:

- Evaluate each patient to determine if he or she has the potential to abuse the prescribed opioids.

- Discuss the risk versus the benefit of opioid treatment with your patients.

- If opioid treatment is ideal, start at the lowest doses.

- Ensure that the prescriptions you write do not exceed 90 morphine milligram equivalents per day, for greater than seven days. Also make sure they are extended-release or long-acting opioids and that they are not prescribed in combination with other therapies.

- Look for alternative treatments for patients with chronic pain.

Please pay close attention to the following example, especially if you are a person with an addictive personality. This real-life example is about a dear friend of mine, Deb, who found herself deep in the clutches of drug abuse.

Deb's Testimony

I have a testimony of using mindfulness in the beginning of my recovery process. Here is part of my testimony of how God does what He does supernaturally.

My dilemma was serving God while using crack cocaine for seventeen years, but I began using drugs and alcohol at age thirteen. I went to see a psychiatrist, who referred me to partial hospitalization for three weeks. While I was in a group, a woman was teaching dialectical behavior therapy (DBT) skills to stay in the moment and practice mindfulness. She told me I have control over my thoughts. That is the first I ever heard of that. But I was willing to do whatever it is to get through this psychotic state of thinking.

I was diagnosed with major depressive disorder. I was still using at that time. I was prescribed medicine to stop the racing thoughts. I took it, and that day it worked immediately to slow my thought process. Every time I thought of crack, I said, "The blood of Jesus." The thought of crack at first was so intense that I immediately could only say "Jesus." Little did I know how powerful that was. Within the first month of being in there, my use decreased. That was in July 2009. My last use was on October 9, 2009.

I went into outpatient treatment and was put into a DBT class. That is where the fire of the Holy Spirit replaced all the years the enemy stole out of my life with the gift of wisdom and knowledge. This is when God supernaturally transformed my thinking within weeks. My therapist, who taught the class, was blown away by the immediate change.

She taught us how to be mindful of ourselves and our surroundings and said that doing so can trigger us, so she taught us the skill of meditation, or being in the moment. I was being in the moment with God. I would look at a particular object for five minutes and repeatedly say, "Jesus. Jesus. Jesus." I would go outside to focus on a tree for five minutes, and when my thought process would start running away again, I would bring it back to the tree. I looked at everything on the tree that God designed. Every new thought was God.

One day, I was asked to attend a teaching that my girlfriend was doing, and when I heard what she was teaching on, it blew me away. She was teaching on Dr. Caroline Leaf! I stood up and shouted out, "I am a walking testimony of her teachings!" God taught me what she teaches. Blown away at this point, I immediately contacted Dr. Leaf's team, and they sent me, as a gift, her books and a CD. That was in 2010. Need I say anymore of how our relationship has evolved? Today I am blessed to have the honor of telling you this all because of the seed God placed in me.

In this testimony, Deb gave us a short version of how powerful our minds are. We can choose either God's mind and way of doing things or something less. She demonstrates the former.

Please remember that dopamine is a pleasure-reinforcement brain-and-gut chemical that we make internally. Choosing mental, emotional, and physical activities that elevate dopamine in your brain is important. We can make choices that cause increased brain levels of dopamine without ever having to take medication. Dopamine levels are low when we are depressed or sick or with certain neurodegenerative disorders. Antidepressant medication, substance abuse, and alcohol and illicit drug use can also increase dopamine. The correct responses to increase dopamine levels include eating certain vegetables, exercising, laughing, doing things that remind you of good times, and spending time with God. We are meant to be addicted to love, God's character—not synthetic harmful substances or actions. We must choose life-building activities. We also must do the following:

1. Know that God loves us.

2. Know God's intention—that is, His prescription for us.

3. Elevate our thinking, even in the darkness.

4. Confess the light.

For I know the thoughts that I think toward you, saith the LORD, thoughts of peace, and not of evil, to give you an expected end (Jer. 29:11, KJV).

Don't deny circumstances. Instead, acknowledge the problem or bad report so that you have a *name* that Jesus will work on. After that, call *Jesus's name* and claim promises for yourself and about that area. See yourself prospering in that area, and continue to confess His Word on that subject. Proclaim it in Jesus's name. God thoughts will replace fear. The joy and peace that only Jesus can give through the Holy Spirit will replace and overwhelm negative thoughts and feelings. This changes the chemical communication of the hypothalamus to the other systems. The body has to respond as you use your soul (mind, will, and emotions) like a surgeon's scalpel—that is, precisely, focusing on His life-giving words. God's thoughts as expressed as His words are released. All evil has to be annihilated!

My friend, Deb, did exactly what I described, and God brought His "A" game to knock out and replace one of the most difficult afflictions anyone can experience: addiction. She had a disordered mind, body dependency, and a weak spirit-state. All three areas were in bad condition. However, in acknowledging Jesus by just saying His name, she initiated a chain reaction in all three areas of her being. She allowed God to get in the center of her being by a willful act, a decision. This purposeful decision created a cascade of spiritual, emotional, and ultimately physical and chemical effects in her brain and nervous system/ stem cells, which led to transformation!

Don't tell me God doesn't love us. He uses a decision to transform all three parts of who we are that are all intimately connected.

God's prescription, in summary, is that He is a promise-keeper and way-maker for those who know Him and accept His help.

Let's take God at His Word!

Cancer

Cells are the basic units that make up the human body. Cells grow and divide to make new cells as the body needs them. Usually, when cells get too old or damaged, they die. Then new cells take their place.

Cancer begins when genetic changes impair this orderly process. Cells start to grow uncontrollably. These cells may form a mass called a *tumor*. A tumor can be malignant (cancerous) or benign (not cancerous). Cancerous tumors grow and spread to other parts of the body, while benign tumors remain in one location. They might grow, but they do not spread.

Doctors categorize cancer into types based on where it began. Four main types of cancer are as follows:

1. **Carcinomas**—*Carcinomas* are the most common type of cancer. A carcinoma begins in the skin or the tissue that covers the surface of internal organs and glands. Carcinomas usually form solid tumors. Examples include prostate cancer, breast cancer, lung cancer, and colorectal cancer.

2. **Sarcomas**—A *sarcoma* begins in the tissues that support and connect the parts of the body. A sarcoma can develop in fat, muscles, nerves, tendons, joints, blood or lymph vessels, cartilage, or bone.

3. **Leukemias**—*Leukemia* is a cancer of the blood. It begins when healthy blood cells change and grow uncontrollably. The four main types of leukemia are acute lymphocytic leukemia, chronic lymphocytic leukemia, acute myeloid leukemia, and chronic myeloid leukemia.

4. **Lymphomas**—*Lymphoma* is a cancer that begins in the lymphatic system, which is a network of vessels and glands that help fight infection. There are two main types of lymphomas: Hodgkin lymphoma and non-Hodgkin lymphoma. Hodgkin lymphoma (Hodgkin disease) is a cancer that starts in white blood cells called *lymphocytes*, which are part of the body's immune system.

As a cancerous tumor grows, the bloodstream or lymphatic system can carry cancer cells to other parts of the body. During this process, known as *metastasis*, the cancer cells grow and might develop into new tumors. One of the first places a cancer often spreads is to the lymph nodes. *Lymph nodes* are tiny, bean-shaped organs that help fight infection. They are in clusters in different parts of the body, such as the neck, groin area, and under the arms.

Cancer can also spread through the bloodstream to distant parts of the body, including the bones, liver, lungs, or brain. Even if the cancer spreads, it is still named for the area where it began. For example, if breast cancer spreads to the lungs, it is called metastatic breast cancer, not lung cancer.

We control our minds and the limbic system and circuit of Papez, those structures in our brains that serve as interfaces with our bodies. These structures affect the four trillion cells in our bodies and affect the immune system, for good or bad. There is voluminous research about how we can use the immune system to kill cancer. Even in my field of brain surgery, immune mechanisms are being used to kill cancer. The human immune system is activated or deactivated from our thinking. We can, therefore, have better outcomes by thinking positive thoughts than by taking medications and undergoing laboratory manipulation of those cells outside the body to be put back inside the body to do what they were meant to do. If we correctly believe that God will heal our bodies and rid us of cancer, then those systems will be activated as God intended and will kill cancer cells. If we incorrectly believe we are doomed to die, then those systems will facilitate cancer growth.

The 700 Club featured the story of a woman named Shirley Williams who was diagnosed with stage IV cancer in 2012. It had spread from her breast to her bones, organs, and lymph nodes. Her doctor told her she had about ninety days to live, after undergoing conventional therapies. Shirley was in great pain and so weak that she could barely walk. She was tempted to give in and just lie down and die.[17] But then she and her husband decided to fight her cancer with faith. Shirley said, "I never found one place in the Scriptures where someone came to Jesus for healing that they were not healed. I began to see that faith was not just believing that God was *able*, but it was believing that He *will*."[18]

Shirley's doctor advised her to sweat. So she began detox, saunas, and exercise. She began eating organic foods, and her

17. Zsa Zsa Palagyi, "Stage IV Cancer Healed!" CBN, *The 700 Club*, http://www1.cbn.com/stage-iv-cancer-healed.
18. Ibid

husband commanded the pain to cease in the name of Jesus. Three months later, a PET scan showed that the tumors were gone, and there was no evidence that there was cancer in her body. Shirley's doctor said, "I believe that when a person has stage IV cancer and the cancer is gone, it's a miracle."[19]

This is another example of how much God loves us by putting these healing mechanisms and cells into our bodies. All we must do is believe His promises for us, state those promises until we believe that they are true for us individually, and believe there is no truth above those truths from God. We cast the other thoughts down, and this will create the desired healing cascade that God has planned for us every time!

> Casting down imaginations, and every high thing that exalteth itself against the knowledge of God; and bringing into captivity every thought to the obedience of Christ (2 Corin. 10:5, KJV).

There are many stories like this of people refusing to believe cancer will destroy them. They claim God's promise of healing, and they surprise their doctors and everyone else when the cancer disappears from their bodies.

Stroke

A stroke is sometimes called a "brain attack." It happens when blood flow is cut off to an area of the brain, and brain cells are deprived of oxygen and begin to die. When brain cells die during a stroke, abilities controlled by that area of the brain such as memory and muscle control are lost.

---

19. Ibid

According to the National Stroke Association, stroke is the fifth- leading cause of death in the United States. Each year, nearly 800,000 people experience a new or recurrent stroke. A stroke happens every forty seconds, and every four minutes, someone dies from stroke. And stroke is the leading cause of adult disability in the United States.[20]

Jerry Savelle is president of Jerry Savelle Ministries International. He has written more than seventy books and has taught in more than three thousand churches in twenty-six nations.

In the fall of 2016, Savelle underwent routine surgery to remove the plaque in his carotid artery, which was blocking blood flow to his brain. During the surgery, he had a stroke. He lost the use of his right arm and suffered memory loss. He couldn't remember his daughters' names, Scriptures, or the names of everyday objects.[21]

Every day, he spent time reading the Word and listening to the sermons of great spiritual teachers. Then he remembered the first message he ever preached at a Kenneth Copeland meeting. It was a message from Matthew 8, about a centurion who came to Jesus, saying, "My servant lies at home paralyzed, suffering terribly." When Jesus offered to go to his home to heal his servant, the soldier said he didn't deserve to have Jesus in his home. The centurion continued, "But just say the word, and my servant will be healed" (from Matthew 8:5–8).[22]

---

20. "What Is Stroke?" National Stroke Association, http://www. stroke.org/understand-stroke/what-stroke.

21. Jerry Savelle Ministries International, https://www.jerrysavelle. org/partner-letter-december-2016/.

22. Ibid

Savelle writes, "I've preached it now for almost forty-eight years, but I have a new appreciation for it today—it has literally extended my life. Solomon was right when he said that the Word is 'Life unto those that find them and health to all their flesh" (Prov. 4:23). The literal Hebrew says, 'Medicine to their flesh.' The more Word you put into your spirit, the greater the effect it'll have on your flesh!"[23]

Reverend Savelle described his stubborn determination to accept the brain healing that was due him since Jesus took the stripes of disease for him on the whipping post and when He wore the bloody crown of thorns as it was jammed into His skull and brain, thereby exchanging any brain issue or mind/emotional pathology for us, as long as we believe in the exchange He made for us. We get His pure sound mind and brain in the healed state in exchange for our sicknesses and diseases in our brains and minds.

Reverend Savelle was discharged after his hospital stay without the ability to use his hand to turn the doorknob, much less remember how to turn on and ride any item in his extensive motorcycle and car collection. He walked from the house to the garage that stored his automobiles. He thought that although he couldn't remember how to turn on or ride the vehicles, still "I am going to turn them on before leaving this garage." And he did exactly what he set his mind to do. His strong spirit told his mind what to do, which activated neural stem cells in his brain to repair any damaged dysfunctional brain tissue. He left that garage the same day with complete return of practical and motor memory of how to ride and turn on those vehicles. Also, his hand strength had improved during that short walk

23. Ibid

from the garage to his house. He could now use his formerly paralyzed hand to open the door!

Given this example, you can't convince me that God is not thoughtful to us. He created each of us from two stem cells (egg and sperm) in our mothers' wombs. He put all the healing mechanisms into those two cells that would grow into trillions of cells. Their complex functions can be influenced and activated by thoughts and emotions so that we may live a repaired, whole life in the face of emotional, psychological, or physical damage. These mechanisms are far too complex to just occur by chance. As a neurosurgeon who sees hundreds of different kinds of strokes, I can tell you that the miracle that occurred in Reverend Savelle's brain thanks to his strong spirit and mind is the ultimate testament to God's love for us and His applied brilliance. Science is only a language that God uses to help us explain a little of how He does what he does. It is not *opposed* to what He does. People try to get credit for "discovering" what He has already created.

Savelle's recovery is a wonderful example of how we can activate the healing mechanisms that God put in us when our bodies are damaged.

Traumatic Brain Injuries

It was once believed that the condition known as *chronic traumatic encephalopathy* (CTE) afflicted primarily boxers. It is a progressive degenerative disease that afflicts the brains of people who have suffered repeated concussions and traumatic brain injuries, such as athletes who take part in contact sports and members of the military.

The brain of an individual who suffers from CTE gradually deteriorates and will eventually lose mass. Certain areas of the brain are particularly liable to atrophy, though other areas are prone to becoming enlarged.

Dr. Bennet Omalu is a physician, forensic pathologist, and neuropathologist who was the first to discover and publish findings of CTE in American football players while working at the Allegheny County Coroner's Office in Pittsburgh. Today, he is a professor at the University of California, Davis, Department of Medical Pathology and Laboratory Medicine.

While performing brain autopsies on many high-profile sports professionals, Dr. Omalu noted specific proteins caused by repeated impacts to the brain that manifested in depression, self-destructive behaviors, and incidents of domestic violence.

As with all patients, we must treat patients who have CTE with God's prescription and remind them of His love and the potential for mind renewal by reading His Word. We need to administer the appropriate care that covers all three realms of each individual. Only God knows people from the inside out. He knows their thoughts and who they really are.

He can lead the treating physician or clinician in a way that an ideal solution will be applied for that specific individual.

God also leads Dr Caroline Leaf, a highly respected cognitive neuroscientist, in treating people with all types of brain injuries. He gave her an idea that later became a system to help people heal their brains and minds. She began her career in academics and clinical work. She now travels the world teaching people how to use their minds to overcome physical or mental obstacles.

Multiple Sclerosis

When someone has an infection, cancer, or allergic reactions, one of the main components that exists in their bloodstream, as part of their immune system, is *cytokines*. As mentioned earlier, cytokines are immunoregulatory proteins (such as interleukin or interferon) that are secreted by cells, especially of the immune system.

The effects of central inflammatory processes may account for some of the behavioral symptoms seen in multiple sclerosis (MS) patients, which cannot be explained by psychosocial factors or the CNS damage hypothesis. This immune mediated hypothesis is supported by indirect evidence from experimental and clinical studies on the effect of cytokines on behavior, in which peripheral as well as central cytokines may cause depressive symptoms. There are emerging clinical data from MS patients to provide support for an association of central inflammation (as measured by MRI) as well as inflammatory markers with depressive symptoms and fatigue.[24]

In one study of patients who had been treated for multiple sclerosis (MS), one group was composed of patients who were being treated were doing well on their medications and had no problems. The other group of MS patients was being treated, but they experienced more emotional trauma in their lives than the patients in the first group.

------

24. Stefan M. Gold, PhD, and Michael R. Irwin, MD, "Depression and Immunity: Inflammation and Depressive Symptoms in Multiple Sclerosis," *Immunology and Allergy Clinics of North America 29*, no. 2 (May 2009): 309–20, https://www.sciencedirect.com/science/article/pii/S0889856109000095?via%3Dihub.

The researchers found that the cytokines were higher in the group of MS patients who had more psychological issues. We also see increased cytokines when the body has inflammation. We see them heavily in cancer and in immune disorders. This shows that there is a correlation between what we think and our physiology. I think it's important to take a broader, more longitudinal view to really appreciate this concept.

Psoriasis

A team of researchers in New York points to "an explosion of scientific advancements showing the close interconnection between the central and the peripheral nervous, the immune, and the endocrine systems." Ongoing translational studies report that the discipline of psychoneuroimmunology may be of significant relevance to the generation and evolution of human diseases, including cutaneous ones such as psoriasis.[25]

Researchers noted that numerous psychosocial interventions aimed at the reduction of stress have proved to be successful for the treatment of psoriasis (as well as psychological symptoms). Hypnosis is one alternative therapy with evidence of utility for these patients. Psoriasis patients improved significantly during hypnosis sessions, in which they received suggestions that they were being exposed to "whatever they believed...would ameliorate their condition." More traditional therapies have also been applied with some success to patients with psoriasis. One study showed that a short program of cognitive behavioral

25. J. Moynihan, E. Rieder, and F. Tausk,
"Psychoneuroimmunology: The Example of Psoriasis," University of Rochester and New York University, *Ginorale Italiano di Dermatologia e Venereologia 145*, no. 2 (April 2010): 221–8.

therapy (CBT) was associated with a decrease in the number and frequency of psoriasis symptoms reported even six months following the program's end. (It should be noted that this was not a randomized control trial [RCT]; patients were allowed to choose CBT.)[26]

Psychotherapy—including stress reduction and imagery—was also shown to have a positive effect on disease activity. Also, in a very small group of randomized subjects, meditation resulted in improvement of psoriatic lesions, and the addition of imagery to meditation had no added effect. In another study, the addition of mindfulness-based stress-reduction tapes during the time that the psoriasis patients were inside phototherapy booths markedly accelerated the time to clearance of the psoriasis plaques when compared to patients who received phototherapy without the tapes. This study demonstrates that brief psychosocial interventions may not only result in an enhanced overall well-being of the patients but can specifically improve the psoriatic disease itself.[27]

The Battle Against Illness Is Won in Our Minds

Drug addiction is born from real and perceived negative experiences that translate into emotional energy that drives the formation of our personalities, joys, and fears. Those experiences affect our spirits (the real "us"), our souls (mind, will, and emotions), and our bodies. Studies have shown that chronic stress leads to depression and adulthood illnesses, as well as addictions.

---

26. Ibid.

27. Ibid

Addictions and other health issues originate squarely from the "battlefield of the mind." Joyce Meyer is a Charismatic Christian author, speaker, and the president of Joyce Meyer Ministries in Missouri. For years, she has been laying the foundation for this concept and introducing the world to mindfulness. In her best-selling book *Battlefield of the Mind*, she offers strategies for dealing with the thousands of thoughts you think every day and explains how to focus the mind the way God thinks.

Throughout this book, I state that we are faced with choices every day that affect our spiritual, mental, and physical health. Joyce Meyer agrees: she says, "Jesus has made arrangements for us to be filled with life by putting His own mind in us. We can choose to flow in the mind of Christ."

One way to do that, she says, is to "learn how to discern life and death." This means that we need to simply be aware when negative thoughts begin to creep into our minds. Here is how she explains this awareness:

> Let's say I'm thinking about an injustice I suffered because of another person, and I begin to get angry. I start thinking about how much I dislike that individual. If I am discerning, I will notice that I am being filled with death. I am getting upset, tense, stressed out—I may even be experiencing physical discomfort. Headache, stomach pain, or undue fatigue may be the fruit of my wrong thinking. On the other hand, if I am thinking how blessed I am and how good God has

been to me, I will also discern that I am being filled with life.[28]

Mindfulness: A Healing Strategy

Mindfulness can be an effective way to relax the mind and ease stress. I describe it as an inward self-reflective mental posture. It's "focused relaxation." Mindfulness with a God focus is an emotional posture of appreciation for God's creation in you that develops patience. This mental exercise does not oppose the things of God, just like yoga—a physical exercise in relaxation—doesn't oppose God, either.

In his book *Full Catastrophe Living*, scientist and meditation teacher Jon Kabat-Zinn discusses a hundred or so scientific studies suggesting that our thoughts, emotions, and life experiences influence our health. He says the practice of *mindfulness*—moment- to-moment awareness and cultivating an attitude of non-striving and non-doing—can bolster our immune systems, determine which genes in our chromosomes are turned on, lower blood pressure, regulate emotions under stress, reduce pain, increase our stamina, and make us much more fun to be around.[29]

Kabat-Zinn launched a Mindfulness-Based Stress Reduction (MBSR) course that is offered through the Stress Reduction Clinic at the University of Massachusetts Medical Center in

---

28. Joyce Meyer, *Battlefield of the Mind: Winning the Battle in Your Mind* (New York: Warner Books, 1995), 162.

29. Therese J. Borchard, "Mind Your Health: Using Mindfulness to Heal Your Body," PsychCentral, https://psychcentral.com/blog/mind-your-health-using-mindfulness-to- heal-your-body/.

Worcester, Massachusetts. More than twenty thousand people have taken the course. As of 2013, there were more than 720 mindfulness-based programs modeled on MBSR in hospitals, medical centers, and clinics across the United States and worldwide. Kabat-Zinn describes the course as an "intensive self-directed training program in the art of conscious living."[30]

He explains that we cannot eliminate stress from our lives, and running from it or trying to numb ourselves from stress-related problems with drugs and alcohol simply creates more problems. Instead, he says we need to learn to live with the inevitable stressors of life by embracing mindfulness, which he says is the art that involves "learning to see ourselves and the world in new ways, learning to work in new ways with our bodies and our thoughts and feelings and perceptions, and learning to laugh at things a little more, including ourselves, as we practice finding and maintaining our balance as best we can."[31]

Researchers at the University of Wisconsin looked at the effects of Kabat-Zinn's course that was delivered in a corporate setting during working hours with healthy but stressed-out employees. The researchers found that brain scans of those who participated in the course showed activity suggesting they were handling negative emotions like anxiety and frustration more effectively (or in a more emotionally intelligent way) than the group that was on the waiting list for the course. There was right-sided to left-sided movement within the prefrontal cerebral cortex that is involved in the expression of emotions.

---

30. Jon Kabat-Zinn, *Full Catastrophe Living: Using the Wisdom of Your Body and Mind to Face Stress, Pain, and Illness* (New York: Bantam Books, 2013), xlviii.

31. Ibid, liv.

The study also found that the people who completed the eight-week training in mindfulness showed a significantly stronger antibody response in their immune systems after being given a flu vaccine (at the end of the eight weeks of training) than did those who were on the waiting list.[32]

Another study conducted at UCLA and Carnegie Mellon University showed that participating in an MBSR program reduced expression of genes related to inflammation, measured in immune cells sampled from blood draws. The mindfulness training also lowered C-reactive proteins in participants, which is an indication of inflammation—a core element of many diseases.[33]

Kabat-Zinn's mindfulness training and Dr. Caroline Leaf's "Switch on Your Brain" program, with a five-step learning process, are compelling examples of the ways in which we can lead individuals to learn how to cope with stress. But to make mindfulness truly beneficial to our tri-part makeup, we must focus on God during those moments of silence. If you will use this easy strategy to take advantage of your God- given mechanisms for healing, you can learn to cope with stress in healthy ways and to learn valuable lessons from the difficulties that we encounter throughout life.

How to Practice Mindfulness and Communication with Our Creator

It is a testament to God's love for us that He has given us the ability to relieve our own suffering simply by being mindful.

---

32. Borchard, PsychCentral.
33. Ibid.

Mindfulness involves simply being still, becoming aware of your environment, focusing on your breathing, and reining in your wandering mind. Its observing God's physical plan in how He has uniquely created you. You are more aware of and are taking a conscious moment to peruse God's orchestra of life in you. Here are some basic instructions for practicing mindfulness. Every mindfulness coach states these instructions slightly differently.

1. **Sit in a comfortable position.** Find a place to sit that feels calm and quiet. Sit cross-legged in an upright position if you can, but don't assume a rigid posture.

2. **Rest your eyes gently on the floor in front of you, or close them.** Focus on a spot about four to six feet away. If you are closer to the wall than that, let your gaze rest on the wall wherever it lands. You can listen to the tempo of the Lord's voice when your eyes are closed as well.

3. **Focus on your body and the environment around you.** When your attention wanders away, gently bring it back to your body and the environment. Now focus on God's love for you. Think about how He created you in His own image, with mechanisms for healing in every part of your soul, mind, and body. Quietly ask God to allow you to know His heart. Acknowledge that God loved us all enough to send His only Son to die on the cross for our sins. Praise Him and thank Him for all He has done for you.

4. **Just breathe.** Focus on your breathing as you take in air and release air from your lungs. Pray in your heavenly language. Listen to the cadence of the prayer

language. Be aware of how it changes, including when you sing it. Notice how much lighter you feel as the Lord lifts those burdens off your shoulders. When you notice that you have gotten so caught up in thoughts that you have forgotten that you're sitting in the room, gently bring yourself back to your breath and speaking in your heavenly language. Try not to time yourself. Be led by the Holy Spirit regarding the amount of time in prayer. Often, we get restless early on in our walk with the Lord, until we experience the joy that comes from being in His presence. Think about all the miracles that God has performed in your life and the lives of others. You'll soon begin to pray longer and not pay attention to your time with the Lord. This will allow you to relax mentally and physically. You will be filled with more peace and joy each time you commune with the Lord.

It takes practice to learn to sit quietly and to return your wandering mind to focus on the current moment and your surroundings. Likewise, listening to the Holy Spirit's voice takes effort to develop when you are relaxed and quiet. Read Scripture and pray in tongues to build up your spirit. This requires a focused heart to develop a mature "spiritual ear."

Focusing on God Changes Our Minds

It is extremely beneficial to focus on God and His love for us, whether or not we are engaged in mindfulness meditation. Focusing on God as we go about our daily activities fills our minds with positive thoughts, optimism about the future, and gratitude for the blessings He has bestowed on us. Often, people view God as a judgmental, angry God who is ready to pounce on any mistake or misstep we make, like a judgmental five-year-old child. He is not at all that. He loves us. We knock, and He answers out of love and concern for our future! God loves us, wants to bless us, and hears us cry out to Him.

> The eyes of the Lord are upon the righteous, and his ears are open unto their cry (Ps. 34:15, KJV).

Whether we are praying, singing hymns of praise, reading His Word, listening to Christian music, speaking in tongues, or engaging in fellowship with other Christians, that focus on God can change our minds in a good way and break that loop of negative thoughts, which we'll discuss in chapter 3.

Research proves this to be true.

Herbert Benson, MD, is a cardiologist, a professor of medicine at the Medical School of Harvard University, and the founder of the Mind/ Body Medical Institute at Massachusetts General Hospital in Boston. For the past thirty-five years, he has conducted studies on prayer.

Dr. Benson believes there is a relationship between prayer and health. He says, "We found that there is a link between the physical condition of a person and any repeated activity of concentration he does, which involves control over random thoughts. Most people make it through prayer. So, we believe that when a person repeats a prayer over and over again, it can help cure a disease, especially if it is caused by stress."[34]

---

34. "Dr. Herbert Benson: Prayer Has a Healing Effect," Learning Mind, https://www.learning-mind.com/ dr-herbert-benson-prayer-has-a-therapeutic-effect/.

Dr. Benson has studied people who prayed repeatedly and were very focused during the prayer. The magnetic resonance imaging showed that there was a decrease in metabolism, heart rate, blood pressure, breathing rate, and brain activity. He states, "Thus, we got scientific proof that prayer affects body functions and fights stress."[35]

Researchers studying HIV patients found that religious attendance (attending church) was associated with a 50 percent reduction in the likelihood of HIV viremia. Researchers concluded that reported church attendance at the time of entry into HIV care is associated with viral load suppression at twelve months. This finding may help explain why HIV patients who are more involved in religious/spiritual practices have longer survival with the disease.[36]

Those HIV patients' immune systems were activated because God set it up that way. When people pray, the autoimmune system is activated, and the benefits go far beyond what medication does. Again, God created us with the ability to heal from the time we were two cells old. This shows how much He loves us.

Speaking in tongues can aid in healing, too. Studies suggest that people who speak in tongues rarely suffer from mental problems. A recent study of nearly one thousand evangelical Christians in England found that those who engaged in the

---

35. Ibid.

36. "Religious Attendance and Viral Load in HIV," *Crossroads Newsletter of the Center for Spirituality*, Duke University, October 2016, https://spiritualityandhealth.duke.edu/ images/pdfs/CSTH_ Newsletter_Oct_2016.pdf.

practice were more emotionally stable than those who did not.[37]

Researchers at the University of Pennsylvania took brain images of five women while they spoke in tongues and found that their frontal lobes—the thinking, willful part of the brain through which people control what they do—were relatively quiet, as were the language centers.

The regions involved in maintaining self-consciousness were active.[38] The language area in the frontal lobes of the brain is normally activated when singing, talking, or doing nonverbal communication. When you sing and pray intensely, those areas light up. But when you speak in tongues, none of it lights up!

Why is that? People who speak in tongues are making a wonderful noise, and everyone can hear it, but they aren't using their brains to create the noise. So it can't be due to any structure in the body. If it were, it would show up on the imaging. That means the spirit is controlling it! That is scientific proof that praying in tongues has a spiritual, mental, and physical effect.

> And when Paul laid his hands on them, the Holy Spirit came on them, and they *began* speaking in [unknown] tongues (languages) and prophesying (Acts 19:6, AMP).

37. Benedict Carey, "A Neuroscientific Look at Speaking in Tongues," *The New York Times*, November 7, 2006, https://www.nytimes.com/2006/11/07/health/07brain.html.
38. Ibid.

Now, some people have grown up in churches that neither believe in nor teach the practice of speaking in tongues, the "heavenly language." This is unfortunate. God does not demand that we speak in tongues. But I will tell you this from personal experience: if you do speak in the heavenly language, you will experience a much more powerful bond with your Creator than you possibly can without doing so. By the way, Satan cannot understand what you are saying when you speak in tongues! We have examples of powerful people in the Bible who spoke in the heavenly language and as a result were preserved in the face of spiritual, emotional, and physical distress to the point of death on multiple occasions. Paul was the perfect example of what he described when he addressed the Church at Corinth.

I thank my God, I speak with tongues more than ye all (1 Corin. 14:18, KJV).

The God Prescription: Strategies to Heal Illness by Focusing on the Tri-Part Human

1. Believe God, make your request known to Him, stand in faith, and watch Him bless you with healing and wholeness! A little seed sown gives continuous blessing.

2. Be strong in Spirit first so that when your body is weak, you can get through it and become stronger.

3. Build deep relationships with Jesus Christ and with the people around you.

4. Confess your sins to God, and ask for forgiveness.

5. Forgive people who have wronged you.

6. Practice stress-reduction techniques like deep breathing, visualizing positive scenarios, listening to pleasant music, and praising God.

7. To alleviate pain and stress-related issues, practice *mindfulness*—moment-to-moment awareness and cultivating an attitude of non-striving and non-doing. Remember that God created these relaxation mechanisms and physiologic responses. He deserves the credit and cannot be taken out of the equation. Any technique without God being acknowledged has no place for us and no lasting effect on our spirits, souls, and bodies. None of these ideas should replace God's methodology or supplant or be uncoupled from Him.

3

Medicine Is Evolving to Treat the Whole Person

The understanding that emotions affect physical health dates as far back as the second-century physician Galen and the medieval physician and philosopher Moses Maimonides. In contrast, modern medicine has largely continued to treat the mind and body as two separate entities. In the past thirty years, however, research focused on the link among health and emotions, behavior, social and economic status, and personality has moved both research and treatment from the fringe of biomedical science into the mainstream.

I believe the mind and body are separate entities. I have personally communicated with patients while I was exposing their brains during surgery. Electrically testing and stimulating patients' brains during neurosurgery gives me a firsthand account of how the brain functions with external stimulation. The brain does not function on its own. It is powered by your spirit, which leverages your soul (mind, will, and emotions) to be an organ that expresses your thoughts through your physical body. As a brain surgeon, I often witness the moment life goes out of a person's body while I am gazing at and touching his or her brain.

Seizures in the physical brain can create laughter but not memories after the seizures or after direct stimulation. This is because the mind is separate from brain matter. The brain matter is the processor that connects the spirit person and his or her mind to the physical world. I have seen patients' consciousness leave their bodies, as if we were turning a light off. This further reinforces my direct observations. Also supporting my assertion that the mind and the brain are separate entities is the fact that people who have compulsive personality disorders can regulate their compulsive disorder if they choose to do so.

Aetna Medicare Solutions Is Getting It Right

The health-care community is just now beginning to add *spirit* to the equation. Recently, Aetna® Medicare Solutions began centering its message to patients around "a total approach to your health and wellness." The health plan's website says, "We understand that health is more than physical. At Aetna we believe in the need to take care of the whole you—body, mind, and spirit. That's why our Medicare plans take a total approach to health, so you can age actively." Medicare Advantage plans cover doctors and hospitalization in one simple plan. They also can include prescription drug coverage, health coaching, mental health programs, transportation to medical appointments, and meals after a hospital stay. The plan assigns qualified patients with a care manager, who assesses their overall health objectives and needs and designs a plan of care to treat "the whole person."[39]

---

39. Aetna Medicare Solutions, https://www.aetnamedicare.com/en/compare-plans-enroll/total-health-wellness.html.

Robert Mirsky, MD, is the vice president of medical operations and chief medical officer for Aetna Medicare Solutions. When he was a young family physician twenty years ago, he made sure his patients were *physically* healthy, focusing on their ailments and the biological factors that made them sick. That's what he learned in medical school. Dr. Mirsky now says health care is no longer about solely focusing on people who are sick, but on engaging people throughout their health journey.[40]

"I've really come to understand the social and environmental factors that have an impact on the health and well-being of the people we serve," he says. "Total health and wellness is at the heart of what you should be looking for. It's why health care professionals today are reaching out to people who are generally healthy and promoting a more holistic approach to health and wellness—body, mind, and spirit."[41]

Medical Schools Traditionally Focused Only on the Pathology of Disease

Dr. Mirsky is paving the way to acceptance of a more comprehensive approach to treating the tri-part human. Given that we have such profound evidence of the cause and effect between stress and disease, why don't more physicians consider the whole person—all three components—during diagnosis

---

40. Christina Joseph, "How to Take a Total Approach to Your Health: A Conversation with Aetna Medicare Chief Medical Officer Dr. Robert Mirsky," Aetna Medicare, https://www.aetnamedicare.com/en/understanding-medicare/use-medicare-plan-whole-health.html.

41. Ibid.

and treatment? Part of the problem lies in the fact that the curriculum used in most medical schools has traditionally focused only on the pathology of disease, or the physical aspects.

As I mentioned earlier, when I was in medical school, we were taught about only the pathology side of things: "Here is the disease process, and here is the chemical reason why the process exists. Lab tests confirm that there is an abnormality, and this is the way we are going to treat it with chemicals or surgery." That's where we left the conversation.

Many scientists who become interested in this field say their efforts to investigate aspects of the mind–body connection have been met with skepticism and even derision from the scientific mainstream.

Esther Sternberg, MD, the rheumatologist and NIH researcher mentioned earlier, had the same experience when she arrived at the NIH in 1980 and studied the strange case of a man who developed severe scleroderma—an autoimmune disease—after taking an experimental epilepsy drug, which raised serotonin levels.

"I wanted to and did pursue the connection between the brain and the immune system in the 1980s with many experiments, but I was told not to, that it would ruin my career," Dr. Sternberg said. "To be taken seriously, I followed the typical scientific route; I didn't talk about emotions and beliefs but instead tried to connect findings in immunology to neuroscience and focused on what neuropeptides change the brain." Discussing how emotions might have an impact on the body was taboo, she said.[42]

---

42. Ibid.

But now we realize that often the etiology of a lot of these processes, including cancer, has an emotional and/or psychological basis. At least the emotional and psychological side of the equation is much larger than we anticipated or wanted to acknowledge.

Furthermore, "a growing number of medical schools are including mind–body medicine in their curricula, and a lot of progress has been made in incorporating mind–body medicine into medical schools' curricula, but we've still got a long way to go," said James Gordon, Clinical Professor at Georgetown University and the founder and director of the Center for Mind–Body Medicine.[43]

Gordon recalled the days when the acceptance of mind–body research and medicine was less widespread. Trained as a psychiatrist, he became interested in the 1970s in what was then called *psychosomatic medicine*. He spent a decade at the National Institute of Mental Health to look for scientific evidence for mind–body medicine techniques. "While there was a feeling that mind–body interventions might be important, there was also anxiety that they might come to overshadow NIMH priorities of psychotherapy and psychopharmacology at the time," Gordon observed. Owing to what he called institutional "ambivalence," early studies were published privately rather than by the NIH.[44]

---

43. Vicki Brower, "Mind–Body Research Moves Towards the Mainstream."

44. Ibid.

Research Supports the Mind–Body Connection

Research is beginning to substantiate the powerful connection between the mind and the body. Research that substantiates the human spirit's role in wellness is not as prevalent, but still, the medical community is beginning to acknowledge that there is more to disease than just pathology.

To understand the significance of some of the research in this area, it's important to understand the role of three hormones that increase and decrease when we are subjected to certain situations: cortisol, adrenaline, and norepinephrine. Here is a brief description of the roles they play in our bodies:

1. **Cortisol** is commonly referred to as the body's stress hormone. It works with certain parts of the brain to control mood, motivation, and fear. Your adrenal glands, which are triangle- shaped organs at the top of the kidneys, make cortisol. The hormone manages how the body uses carbohydrates, fats, and proteins; keeps inflammation down; regulates blood pressure; increases blood sugar, or glucose; controls the sleep/wake cycle; boosts energy so we can handle stress; and restores balance after a person experiences stress.

2. **Adrenaline** activation is commonly known as the "fight or flight" hormone. Sometimes called "epineph-rine," it is produced by the adrenal glands after receiving a message from the brain that a stressful situation has presented itself. It is largely responsible for the immediate reactions we feel when stressed. It tells us when we might need to flee a dangerous situation, and it heightens our awareness.

3. **Norepinephrine** plays a similar role to adrenaline. Its primary function is to make us more aware, awake, and focused. It helps shift blood flow away from areas where it isn't needed at the moment to parts of the body that do need it, such as the muscles, so you can run from a dangerous situation. It is essentially a backup to adrenaline.

In the United Kingdom, two large-scale epidemiological and medical studies, known as the Whitehall studies, were conducted among civil servants. The second of those studies found that workers in low-level jobs, in which they have high stress and little autonomy, have more than twice the risk of developing metabolic syndrome—a precursor of heart disease and diabetes—compared with employees in higher-level jobs. The first Whitehall study showed that people from this group are also more inclined to die prematurely than colleagues who do less menial, higher-level work.

In these studies, stress was defined as a high level of demand, a low level of control, and little support from coworkers or supervisors. By measuring people's heart rates and cortisol and adrenaline levels, researchers also found that stress affects the autonomic nervous system and neuroendocrine function.

Other recent research showed that acute and chronic psychological stress, related to low socioeconomic status, can increase the risk of heart attack by increasing circulating levels of platelet–leukocyte aggregates. A study from the University of Utah, first presented at the American Psychosomatic Society meeting in March 2006, showed that hardening of the arteries is more frequent in wives when they and their husbands express hostility during marital disagreements, and the condition is more common in husbands when they or their wives act in a controlling way.

The potential of stress reduction and social support as a therapeutic intervention became evident in the late 1980s during a study of women with breast cancer. David Spiegel, MD, director of the Psychosocial Research Laboratory at Stanford University, wanted to determine whether women with metastatic breast cancer who participated in supportive–expressive group therapy had better quality of life and symptom control than those who received only medical treatment. To his and others' surprise, not only did the women have better quality of life and less pain, but they also lived significantly longer.

These unexpected findings triggered a large body of research into mind–body interventions—such as group therapy, stress-reduction techniques, and cognitive-behavioral therapy (CBT)—and whether they can affect survival and pain in cancer, AIDS, and bone-marrow transplant patients. Findings were split between positive and negative for life expectancy. A main focus of research is the relationship between stress and cardiovascular disease, asthma, inflammatory diseases, autoimmune diseases, and cancer, and whether stress reduction can extend patients' lives. One recent study, for example, found that CBT could help to reduce viral load in HIV-positive men treated with highly active antiretroviral therapy. Researchers attributed the improvement to changes in depressed mood. Depression is under study for possible links to a range of inflammatory diseases; several studies show that depression is an emerging risk factor for heart disease.

When we claim God's promises to give us new life in Him, we can reduce our dependence on our own strength and allow Him to provide us with strength.

> The Lord redeemeth the soul of his servants: and none of them that trust in him shall be desolate (Ps. 34:22, KJV).

Dean Ornish, MD, Helped Increase Awareness

An example of how far mind–body medicine has come over the past three decades is the success story of Dean Ornish, MD, Clinical Professor of Medicine at the University of California in San Francisco and founder, president, and director of the Preventive Medicine Research Institute in Sausalito, California.

When Dr. Ornish claimed in the early 1980s that heart disease could be prevented and even reversed with "lifestyle changes"—a combination of a very low-fat vegetarian diet, meditation or yoga, moderate exercise, stress management, and social support—mainstream medicine did not treat his theory seriously until studies confirmed its validity. Today, Dr. Ornish's program has been adopted in many mainstream cardiovascular clinics throughout the United States, and he continues to research whether his program can help prevent heart disease in patients with type 2 diabetes and halt the progression of prostate cancer.

Patient Demands Have Led to Increased Focus on the Whole Person

An increasing number of US medical schools and centers now have departments devoted to mind–body research and some also to mind– body treatment, including Harvard University, Columbia University, the University of California–Los Angeles, and the University of Pittsburgh. This now-interdisciplinary research field, which also includes behavioral medicine, is often called *psychoneuroimmunology* or *psychoendoneuroimmunology*. It incorporates ideas, belief systems, hopes, and desires, as well as biochemistry, physiology, and anatomy.

Several factors have driven this steady growth. The most prominent factor is patients' increasing interest in self-care, wellness, and alternative medicine and their dissatisfaction with the success of allopathic medicine in preventing and treating chronic illnesses. *Allopathic medicine* aims to combat disease by using remedies (such as drugs or surgery) that produce effects that are different from or incompatible with those of the disease being treated.

Even the US Government Has Begun to Understand

The consumer demand for and use of complementary and alternative medicine has also prompted the US government to become involved. In 1992, under pressure from consumers and with the help of Ohio Congressman Tom Harkin, an alternative medicine enthusiast, Congress mandated the National Institutes of Health (NIH) in Bethesda, Maryland, to open an

Office of Alternative Medicine (OAM) and gave it a $2 million budget.[45]

"Not everyone at NIH was happy about this," commented Theodore Brown, historian of medicine at the University of Rochester. But consumer demand was enthusiastic: when OAM was founded, more than one-third of Americans said that they used relaxation techniques and imagery, biofeedback, and hypnosis, and more than 50 percent used prayer as a complementary or alternative therapy."[46]

Since 1992, government funding for mind–body research has increased considerably. In 2005, the NIH's National Center for Complementary and Alternative Medicine (NCCAM) funded more than 1,200 projects at about 260 institutions. Since 2000, its efforts have focused on understanding the mechanisms of action of various mind–body therapies, including the placebo effect. In its new five-year strategic plan, Director Stephen Straus designated additional funding for mind–body research into a range of diseases, including an ongoing clinical trial that is examining the use of meditation for weight loss, health, and well-being enhancement in obese men and women.[47]

Mind–body research in this country also receives significant money from private foundations. Examples include the Fetzer Institute in Kalamazoo, Michigan, which has spent more than $2 million since 2000; the MacArthur Foundation in Chicago, which invested $10 million between 1989 and 1998

---

45. Vicki Brower, "Mind–Body Research Moves Towards the Mainstream."

46. Ibid.

47. Ibid.

in its Network on Mind–Body Interactions; and the John Templeton Foundation in West Conshohocken, Pennsylvania, which funds several programs on spirituality, health, and medicine.[48]

The God Prescription: Strategies to Heal Illness by Focusing on the Tri-Part Human

1. Patients and physicians have advanced the progress of spirit–mind–body research simply by believing in the value of the whole-person approach to health care and creating a demand for it. We all can continue this progress by being vocal about our need and desire for comprehensive health care.

2. As research continues to demonstrate the significant connection of spiritual and mental/emotional health to physical health, we all should investigate treatments beyond the traditional offerings. Cognitive behavioral therapy, stress reduction, and social support can supplement medication and surgery to address underlying causes of physical illnesses effectively

---

48. Ibid.

4

How Our Emotions Impact Our Physical Health

There are many everyday examples of the ways in which our emotions can trigger physical effects. The mind and the brain, through the hypothalamus and the thalamus, create physiologic responses. It happens all day, every day, all the time. But we are not aware of these processes. Your palms might sweat when you are on a job interview or giving a speech, and the same is true for a child who is sent to the principal's office. Or you might develop a stomach ache when you are anxious with fear.

The Limbic System and the Circuit of Papez

Our emotions are governed by the prefrontal cortex, which is the part of the brain that controls reasoning. The prefrontal cortex affects your hypothalamus, which is one of the master glands that will create a physiologic response, either sympathetic or parasympathetic. This response will constrict the blood vessels to parts of your body and cause you to sweat and feel angst.

The *limbic system* is the emotional side of processing in your brain, and the *circuit of Papez* is the side of your brain that controls memory and helps you recall things that have happened to you. It packages, processes, and stores childhood trauma and other memories.

All these processes combine to create a physiologic, or physical, response. It's all connected. The memory structure (circuit of Papez) and emotional structure (limbic system) are connected to external and internal cues and stimuli or events. These structures in our brains form a loop and influence how we process memory. They work with each other to process past experience for future use.

As the circuit of Papez communicates with the limbic system, which includes the hippocampus, the brain senses information and then processes it.

In 1937, the neuroanatomist James Papez demonstrated that emotion is not a function of any specific brain center. Instead, it is a function of a circuit that involves four basic structures, interconnected through several nervous bundles: the hypothalamus with its mamillary bodies, the anterior thalamic nucleus, the cingulate gyrus, and the hippocampus. This circuit, called the circuit of Papez (Papez circuit), is responsible for the central functions of emotion (affect) and its peripheral expressions (symptoms).[49]

---

49. "Theories on the Role of Brain Structures in the Formation of Emotions," Cerebromente, http://www.cerebromente.org.br/n05/mente/teorias_i.htm.

Love Drives Out Fear

> There is no fear in love [dread does not exist]. But
> perfect (complete, full-grown) love drives out fear, be-
> cause fear involves [the expectation of divine] punish-
> ment, so the one who is afraid [of God's judgment] is
> not perfected in love [has not grown into a sufficient
> understanding of God's love]
>
> (1 John 4:18, AMP).

Fear is a powerful emotion. If it isn't controlled, fear can manifest as all kinds of physical ailments in our bodies. But love
overthrows fear. God gives us the ultimate example of how
to overcome fear and anxiety. He acted by thinking of others
first. As a brain surgeon in practice for almost twenty years,
and after operating on tens of thousands of patients, I can tell
you what love and fear look like. But when we focus on God's
love, peace will wash over us and enable us to overcome our
fears.

> Peace I leave with you; My [perfect] peace I give to
> you; not as the world gives do I give to you. Do not
> let your heart be troubled, nor let it be afraid. [Let My
> perfect peace calm you in every circumstance and give
> you courage and strength for every challenge.] (John
> 14:27, AMP).

Again, the limbic system is a structure in our brains that deals
with emotional input and processing, and the circuit of Papez
is a structure that packages and processes memories. These two
systems work with each other to solidify past experience for
future use. We remember past hurts, injustices, and trauma,

and these experiences often get packaged and mislabeled as something we need to remember for self-preservation.

Young, developing minds can magnify a non-threatening situation into a huge problem. Likewise, real trauma that a child experiences gets packaged deep inside these structures and then becomes incorporated into the soul (mind, will, and emotions). We can suffer long-term detrimental consequences if the reasoning part of our brains doesn't put the experience into context and then convert it into useful energy.

The frontal lobe of the brain doesn't fully develop until our mid- to late twenties. Therefore, most experiences up to that point in our lives might not be properly contextualized. When this happens, it leaves a person's spiritual, mental, and emotional life in shambles.

We live irrationally fearful lives when we deny our spiritual, emotional, and physical needs. To deny any of our three-part being due to perceived or actual wronged experiences leaves us in an unsettled state throughout our adult lives. We have not spent enough time required to allow God's global perspective to enable us to reach transformational levels of love for self and others. God gives us comfort, even in the face of death.

> Even though I walk through the [sunless] [a]valley of the shadow of death, I fear no evil, for You are with me; Your rod [to protect] and Your staff [to guide], they comfort and console me. (Ps. 23:4, KJV).

God's love and our love for one another are much more powerful than fear. We need to know this. People are dying for lack of this knowledge. The fear of the Lord is the beginning of knowledge.

My dear, dear friends, if God loved us like this, we certainly ought to love each other. No one has seen God, ever. But if we love one another, God dwells deeply within us, and his love becomes complete in us—perfect love! (1 John 4:11–12, MSG).

When we focus on the love response, we can use our God-given abilities and emotions to heal ourselves and others. Love promotes power in our thinking and a sound mind. We all know what accomplishments and goal achieving "feel" like long after the achievement has passed. This gives us hope for a bright future.

Our Emotions Are Expressed Through Physical Responses

Research has proven the cause-and-effect relationship between emotions and physical reactions. For example, studies have shown that immune-system function plummets in people who are depressed. That tells us there is a correlation between your emotional state and your immunologic state. We also know there is correlation between the immune system and cancerous states, as well as allergies.

When people have multiple drug allergies, there is often a huge psychological component to them. You can become hypersensitive, and if your immune system is not functioning the way it should, you can have physical reactions to drugs, pollen, and other substances based on an emotional etiology. There might be environmental and/or chromosomal etiology as well.

People react to the same stimuli differently. For example, a soldier who has been serving in a war zone for a long time might know the situation isn't as bad as a new soldier perceives it to be. So even though both soldiers are experiencing the same stimuli on a daily basis, they do not have the same physiologic responses.

This is true in the medical world, too. As mentioned earlier, some people faint at the mere sight of blood, whether it's someone else's or their own. But because I have been operating on people for twenty years, the sight of blood doesn't make me anxious or upset. So I will not have the same physiologic response to it as others might. I see blood all day, every day, as I'm helping people. My physiologic response to a bleeding person is, "What is the source of the bleeding? What do I need to do to fix it?" I will grab my surgical tools and, with a clear mind void of stress, begin repairing the wound. I do not feel too much stress; my pulse and blood pressure will not change significantly. But someone who is not accustomed to seeing blood might have a serious physical reaction. In fact, it is so mundane for me to see blood that I have to be cautious that I'm not calloused by someone bleeding.

The stimuli that cause a physical reaction in a person can be either external or internal. Internal stimuli are our own negative thoughts. Someone might feel a little chest pressure and think, "I'm having a heart attack because my dad had a heart attack at this age." That creates a whole host of negative thoughts and could eventually lead to a heart attack.

You can become so stressed out that your cholesterol levels are affected. We know that only 20 percent of cholesterol comes from dietary sources.

Many women are more emotional during certain times of the month because of the menstrual cycle. In this case, there is a physiologic issue that can create a mental state of being, and vice versa. Let's say a woman's husband says something to her that she normally wouldn't think about much. But if she is feeling more emotional than usual because of her menstrual cycle, his comment might upset her a lot. She can decide to succumb to those emotions, or she can choose not to let them affect her. She can think, "Wait a minute. Yes, this is a problem, but I am overreacting. My emotions are through the roof. I choose not to take what he said to me in that way. I know him, and I know that he didn't mean this as an insult. It's my time of the month, and I know I am overreacting. I'm going to bring this thing way down and not let it affect me."

Phobias are another example of physical reactions to emotions. Some people are so afraid of spiders, snakes, or rats that they break out in a cold sweat and tremble when seeing one. We can control our minds to overcome physical responses to stimuli. We can tell ourselves, "I am not afraid of snakes. I am more powerful than a snake, and the chances of my coming across a snake or being hurt by one are small." If we concentrate on facts, we can have a less emotional response than if we allow our fear to take control over our minds.

Some people develop ulcers when they are worried. Maybe a mother is worried because her son or daughter is serving in the military in a war zone. She can worry so much that she gets ulcers, which eat a hole in her stomach. That is the result of increased production of hydrochloric acid in the stomach. That pathway begins in the mind, which is part of the soul, and then in the brain, which is part of the physical body. The hypothalamus in the brain controls pure sympathetic reactions, which control the hypogastric plexus, which also supplies hydrochloric acid production in our stomachs. So, again, your brain causes that process through your emotions.

It is important to express our emotions and deal with them properly—in a way that honors God and seeks His guidance and comfort. That will help us heal and lead to a sound, powerful mind. Dr. Caroline Leaf, a global leader on thoughtfulness, has some powerful tools to systematically address these issues in a no-nonsense way. I serve as a global advisor on her integrated mind team of physician and scientists, #teamleaf. Here is what Dr. Leaf says about seeking God's help in controlling our emotions:

> When a thought moves from the non-conscious to the conscious mind and we become aware of it, we feel these emotions. It is in this state of feeling the emotions that we have to reach out to God and ask Him to guide the choices we will make based on the perceptions these feelings generate. If we don't let God control, we will draw on our weak human wisdom and make a bad decision. Emotions are wonderful—when driven by the Savior—but can be torturous when driven by carnal wisdom.[50]

---

50. Dr. Caroline Leaf, "Can We Control Emotions and Feelings?" Dr. Leaf's Blog, October 1, 2014, https://drleaf.com/blog/can-we-control-emotions-and-feelings/.

Physical Symptoms Based on Emotions: White Coat Hypertension

A great example of a physical manifestation of an emotional reaction is "white coat hypertension" or "white coat syndrome." This is a disorder in which a person develops high blood pressure only while in the presence of doctors, who often wear white coats. Hypertension is defined as blood pressure readings over 140/90 when measured by a doctor but lower when measured at home. An estimated 15 to 30 percent of people with high blood pressure in the doctor's office have white coat hypertension.

Herbert Benson, MD, is the Director Emeritus of the Benson-Henry Institute (BHI) and the Mind Body Medicine Professor of Medicine at Harvard Medical School. In the late 1960s, Dr. Benson coined the phrase "relaxation response" to describe physiological changes that occur with meditation. As a practicing cardiologist, he observed that many of his patients had high blood pressure at office visits. "On follow-up visits, I found that I had overmedicated them and realized they were experiencing a temporary spike in blood pressure from anxiety—what we came to call 'white coat hypertension,'" Dr. Benson explained.[51]

Intrigued by this observation, he conducted experiments to induce stress and relaxation responses in students. Strangely enough, this was in the same room at Harvard, in which, sixty years before, physiologist and neurologist Walter Cannon had uncovered a direct relationship between stress and neuroendocrine responses in animals—the "fight or flight" response. "I

---

51. Vicki Brower, "Mind–Body Research Moves Towards the Mainstream."

found that the relaxation response was a physiological package, like the 'fight or flight' response," Dr. Benson said.

Practitioners of transcendental meditation asked Dr. Benson to study their meditative states. "I had to bring them round late at night and had to keep my practice separate from my research," Benson said, so that his colleagues did not see his experiments. He found the same response in the mediators as the relaxation response.

On a personal note, as I mentioned earlier, the Lord told me that He wanted me to become a neurosurgeon around the same time that Dr. Benson published his work on the relaxation response.

Dr. Benson noted that public acceptance of the mind–body concept came many years before science acknowledged it: "I was *persona non grata* for a long time and was reprimanded heartily when I published my popular book [on the relaxation response] in 1975," he writes. But in 1994, the work had finally progressed far enough for Dr. Benson to establish the Mind/Body Medical Institute at Harvard University. He explained that mind–body medicine provides one aspect—self-care—of a three-legged model of medicine, which also includes pharmacology and surgery. "The average doctor does not prescribe meditation, breathing exercises, or yoga, and this needs to change," he said.[52]

---

52. Ibid.

Emotion-Related Diseases Are Being Diagnosed More Frequently

As early as the second grade, some children suffer from anxiety, depression, attention deficit hyperactivity disorder (ADHD), and behavioral disorders. These conditions are pleas for help, manifesting as physical conditions. These issues affect children's school work, their ability to make friends, and their physical well-being.

There has been a rise in ADHD diagnoses and other psychological diagnoses that are connected to emotional outpourings in children. Between 2008–09 and 2012–13, visits to a community-based physician that involved an ADHD diagnosis increased by 18.5 percent among children ages five to eighteen—from 93.1 to 110.3 visits per thousand. Nearly 9 percent of all youth visits to community-based physicians during 2012–13 involved a prescription for ADHD medication.[53]

I know for certain that many children who are diagnosed with ADHD do not actually have ADHD. When teachers or parents suspect that a child has ADHD, they will lobby their physicians to have medication such as Ritalin or Adderall prescribed, and they will put the child in remedial classes and behavior-modification sessions. A lot of parents don't want to deal with the behavior problems, and they aren't patient enough to investigate the root cause, so they mislabel their kids. This can be just as damaging as if the child really did have ADHD.

---

53. Dr. David Rabiner, "Study: Rates of ADHD Diagnosis and Medication Treatment Continue to Increase Substantially," SharpBrains, March 22, 2017, https://sharpbrains. com/blog/2017/03/22/study-rates-of-adhd-diagnosis-and-medication-treatment- continue-to-increase-substantially/.

When I was twelve years old, I was diagnosed with ADHD. My mom, an incredibly smart woman, removed a lot of the sugar from my diet. It helped a lot; the sugar I was eating made it difficult for me to focus during class and on my homework assignments. She also realized I was just a super-energetic kid and needed to release energy through physical activity. So she put me in martial arts and swimming.

My mom also realized that my mind was always racing. She encouraged me to do three things at once: I would work on my homework, listen to music, and plan my activities for the next day, all at once. That way, I was able to divide my focus in three areas.

I also came to know the Lord at age twelve. That was a pivotal year for me.

Kids who are three to six years old can't tell you what's going on with them. So it's up to parents, teachers, and clinicians to investigate the root cause of behavioral issues and physical symptoms to find out what's really going on.

Decisions by family members and the medical community about how to cope with children with ADHD have a huge impact on society. Over the past couple of decades, misrepresentation and miscategorization of these diagnoses put us in a bit of quandary as medical professionals. When teachers and others in the school system suspect that there is child abuse or domestic abuse in the home, they often try to assume the role of "savior." They will tell the child, "Johnny, if your parents threaten you in any way with any type of discipline that may be physical, that's bad. You call us. We're the good people who will come to your rescue and save you from the bad parents."

In that scenario, we are setting ourselves up, as a society, for a lot of heartache because most of the discipline and the nurturing come from within the home. There is a parallel between this type of psychology, as it relates to children, and eventual physical diagnosis seen in adults. We are constantly facing moral issues. We are constantly facing more stressors. As the times change, both children and adults are being exposed to more global hurts and injustices, and we don't really know how to handle those. The result is often psychological or emotional trauma, and it manifests itself in physical ways. People attempt to bury trauma that happened to them at a time when their experiences may or may not have been categorized as true trauma.

We Need Each Other

On October 17, 1995, twins Kyrie and Brie were born twelve weeks ahead of their due date. At that time, the standard practice at UMass Memorial Medical Center in Worcester, where the twins were born, was to place them in separate incubators to reduce the risk of infection. So the babies were placed in separate incubators. Kyrie, who weighed 2 lbs. 3 oz., was making good progress and gaining weight, but her tiny sister had breathing and heart-rate problems. She gained little weight, and her oxygen level was low.[54]

On November 12, Brie went into critical condition. Her stick-thin arms and legs turned bluish-gray as she gasped for air. Her

---

54. Steven Ertelt, "Their 'Rescuing Hug' Stunned the World; Now the Twins Are All Grown Up," LifeNews, June 20, 2014, http://www.lifenews.com/2014/06/20/their- rescuing-hug-stunned-the-world-now-the-twins-are-all-grown-up/.

heart rate soared. The parents watched, terrified that their little daughter might die. Nurse Gayle Kasparian, after exhausting all the conventional remedies, decided to try a procedure that was common in parts of Europe but virtually unknown in the United States. With the parents' permission, she placed the twins in the same bed. As soon as she closed the incubator door, Brielle snuggled up to Kyrie and began to calm down. Within minutes, her blood-oxygen readings improved. As she dozed, Kyrie wrapped her left arm around her smaller sister. Brie's heart rate stabilized, and her temperature rose to normal.[55]

That miraculous event has been called "the rescuing hug," and a photo of the twins, with Kyrie's tiny arm wrapped around Brielle, was published in *TIME* magazine and *Reader's Digest*. It has been called "the hug that helped change medicine."[56]

When the twins went home, their parents placed them in the same bed, where they continued to thrive. The twins are now in their late twenties and healthy. Since that time, hospitals have co-bedded hundreds of sets of multiple-birth preemies without a single case of twin-to-twin infection. Clinical studies have shown that premature twins enjoy substantial benefits when they are placed in the same bed together.[57]

What did this demonstrate? That love, closeness, and connection are vital to our physical well-being, whether or not we acknowledge it. We need each other.

---

55. Ibid.

56. Ibid.

57. Ibid.

We Need Emotional Closeness

We need positive feedback. We need emotional closeness. We need affirmation that we're headed in the right direction as we progress through life. Some children, when pushed to over-achieve in areas like piano and mathematics, are often lacking in emotional health if the parents don't give them the emotional closeness, love, and affirmation they need and deserve.

Ted Kaczynski, "the Unabomber," was a domestic terrorist. Between 1978 and 1995, he killed three people and injured twenty-three others in a nationwide bombing campaign that targeted people involved with modern technology. The FBI hunted him for twenty years and captured him in 1996. He is serving a life sentence in Colorado without the possibility of parole.

Kaczynski was a child prodigy in mathematics and entered Harvard College when he was only sixteen. After completing his PhD in mathematics, he taught math at the University of California, Berkeley. He has a high IQ—some reports say 167, others 170. Both are genius scores. But he felt no remorse when he injured or killed people.

According to a *Psychology Today* article, Kaczynski sought treatment for symptoms of depression, anxiety, and sexual-identity confusion when he was a graduate student. He had always been described as "aloof," even as a child, felt emotionally abused by his parents, and was cruelly teased by his peers for being different.[58]

I believe that because he didn't grow up with emotional closeness, he didn't learn to acknowledge that he is a part of this human race or that the entire human race, including him, is of great value. God says that we are valuable.

> So, it is with the one who continues to lay up and hoard possessions for himself and is not rich [in his relation] to God [this is how he fares].

> And [Jesus] said to His disciples, Therefore I tell you, do not be anxious and troubled [with cares] about your life, as to what you will [have to] eat, or about your body, as to what you will [have to] wear.

> For life is more than food, and the body [more] than clothes.

> Observe and consider the ravens: for they neither sow nor reap, which neither have storehouse nor barn; and [yet] God feeds them. Of how much more worth are you than the birds! (Luke12:21–24, AMPC).

No price can be placed on an individual, on a person's worth. When you see yourself in that light, you will also see others in that same light. But if you value yourself less than you should, you will impute that lesser value to others, too.

----

58. Stephen A. Diamond, PhD, "Terrorism, Resentment, and the Unabomber," *Psychology Today*, April 8, 2008, https://www.psychologytoday.com/blog/evil- deeds/200804/terrorism-resentment-and-the-unabomber.

Often, families seem fine to the outside world, but when something drastic happens to an individual, or when he or she commits a horrific crime, we begin to connect the dots. You see that the person was brought up in a dysfunctional home and didn't experience close familial relationships—or worse, suffered abuse at the hands of caregivers.

Then we tend to make huge leaps in logic. We say, "Well, he came from a nice family. I don't know what happened." Nothing has to *happen* to a child, though. Simply failing to receive emotional or spiritual support or guidance can cause abnormal psychological development.

Increasing awareness about the connection among spiritual, mental/ emotional, and physical health hopefully will lead to a greater effort on the part of parents, teachers, coaches, and others to choose their words and actions carefully when interacting with children. We all need to exhibit kindness toward one another and emulate the example God set for us in this regard.

> So, as God's own chosen people, who are holy [set apart, sanctified for His purpose] and well-beloved [by God Himself], put on a heart of compassion, kindness, humility, gentleness, and patience [which has the power to endure whatever injustice or unpleasantness comes, with good temper] (Col. 3:12, AMP).

The God Prescription: Strategies to Heal Your Emotions

1. Love one another. The final component of God's prescription for our spiritual, emotional, and physical ills is that we love Him and love one another. Love is

the ultimate antidote to illness. It's the greatest force, to which every other force must yield.

2. Seek emotional closeness with the people you care about.

3. Recognize the power that words can have on people, especially children. Be kind at all times.

5

The Loop: How The Human Brain Stores Memories

Most of us have negative thoughts playing in our minds on a constant loop, like a CD or an old-time reel of film in a movie projector that never stops, and we aren't even aware of it. That constant negativity is detrimental to our spiritual, mental, and physical health.

Dr. Caroline Leaf is an expert on this topic. She is a world-renowned cognitive neuroscientist with a PhD in communication pathology and is an associate of mine. She specializes in metacognitive and cognitive neuropsychology. Since the early 1980s, she has studied and researched the mind–brain connection. She says 75 to 95 percent of the illnesses that plague us today are a direct result of our thoughts; what we think about affects us physically and emotionally. Here is what Dr. Leaf says about the harm that can result from negative thoughts:

> It's an epidemic of toxic emotions. The average person has over 30,000 thoughts a day. Through an uncontrolled thought life, we create the conditions for illness; we make ourselves sick! Research shows that fear, all on its own, triggers more than 1,400 known

physical and chemical responses and activates more than 30 different hormones. There are intellectual and medical reasons to forgive! Toxic waste generated by toxic thoughts causes the following illnesses: diabetes, cancer, asthma, skin problems, and allergies, to name just a few. Consciously control your thought life, and start to detox your brain! Change in your thinking is essential to detox the brain. Consciously controlling your thought life means not letting thoughts rampage through your mind. It means learning to engage interactively with every single thought that you have, and to analyze it before you decide either to accept or reject it.[59]

No root-cause analysis outside God's Word explains why we develop illnesses of the mind and why the psychological, emotional, and physical ramifications are so significant. Dr. Leaf looks at God's Word, the Bible, through a scientific lens. Her continued work (through books, podcasts, seminars, televised presentations, and teaching) has ushered in a new understanding of how God made our brains and minds to function. Yet we don't take the authority He has given us. We don't use our brains and minds to think deeply and be as impactful in our own realms of influence as we should.

Why Childhood Trauma Can Inflict Lifelong Wounds

As I mentioned before, the prefrontal and frontal lobes of the brain, which enable reasoning, don't fully develop until our

59. Dr. Caroline Leaf, "Controlling Your Toxic Thoughts," Dr. Leaf website, https://drleaf.com/about/toxic-thoughts/.

mid- to late twenties. Therefore, the experiences of young people under the age of twenty might not be properly contextualized. A young person's developing imagination can distort a non-threatening situation into a huge problem.

This is why something that doesn't seem like a big deal to an adult can be a huge deal and traumatic to a child. When we are older, we can look at a situation and use reason to understand why something is occurring and how it is relevant to our lives. Children often carry the traumas they experience with them throughout their lives, and the results can manifest physically. This relative chronology relational example applies to God's view versus our view as little children compared to Him spiritually, intellectually, and emotionally.

Horrific injustices and trauma occur to young people in many homes. And when children remember past hurts, injustices, and trauma, these experiences often get packaged and mislabeled as something they need to remember for self-preservation. Trauma that a child experiences gets packaged deep inside these structures and then becomes incorporated in the soul (mind, will, and emotions). It can have long-term, detrimental consequences if the reasoning part of the child's brain doesn't put the experience into context and then convert it into useful energy.

To deny any of our tri-part being due to our feeling wronged (setting aside the truth of that feeling) leaves us unsettled throughout our adult lives. It can leave our emotional, spiritual, and mental lives in shambles. We often live irrational, fearful lives while denying that our spiritual, emotional, and physical selves require loving connectedness and positive reinforcement.

Satan uses these loops of negative mental processes in an attempt to discourage us and to separate us from God. And it's an effective strategy. We are often quick to believe the worst possible scenario. When something goes wrong, we begin to question our abilities, our relationships, and everything else. We become discouraged and even question God's love for us. We must make a choice to rebuke Satan's attempts to discourage us.

When children receive no affection or human connection, or if the people close to them say negative things to them or treat them badly, those children are likely to develop anxiety and personality issues. Cortisol is released. Then they are likely to grow up to have high blood pressure related to stress. This is true even if a child merely *perceives* to be neglected. Sometimes parents are in a hurry and don't pay attention to a child. If children perceive an unintentional slight as neglect, it will affect them negatively. Any lack of input leads to the same results. Love and appropriate relationships result in a healthy perception of self. This love is delivered in the form of appropriate touch and verbal affirmation. We develop unnatural habits when we don't have appropriate relationships with Mom and Dad, with each other, and especially with God. We all have a desire to be loved and to love. However, if that desire isn't appropriately addressed early in life, then cynicism (iniquity) develops in our hearts. From this lack of appropriate loving relationships as young children, we develop relationships that become destructive physically or emotionally. We then function based on our self-view, which we project inwardly and outwardly.

This neglect, whether real or perceived, can cause psychological damage that leads to low self-esteem, depression, personality disorders, eating disorders, anger, and fear. A child's developing mind tries to make sense of what is occurring before his or her eyes in social environments. These observations are ingredients in the formation of their worldviews and their perspectives about themselves, others, and their Maker.

Negative social experiences (perceived or real) create negative perceptions and thoughts, which then "loop" in our brains and minds from a young age due to external and internal cues and experiences that manifest in all three parts of our existence.

Everyone needs a relationship with Christ to combat the negative effects of the negative loops playing constantly in our minds. The sooner we develop this relationship, the better. Parents would be giving their children the best gift possible by taking them to church starting when they are very young. When they learn that Jesus loves them and that the Word of God contains all the answers to all of life's problems, they will build their own coping strategies that will sustain them for the rest of their lives.

We must focus on God's guidance and promises for our lives. For faith to work, we must believe that He exists and that He loves us. We must know who we are and what tools are available to us. When we do that, we can achieve success in every area of life. *Love and relationships* are at the center of the solution, this prescription from God. They can help us overcome addictions, mental and emotional disorders, autoimmune disorders, high blood pressure, cancer, and other debilitating illnesses and conditions.

Dopamine: The Feel-Good Neurotransmitter

The logo on this truck captures the gut–brain interface.

There are more dopamine receptors in the gut than in the brain!

Dopamine is a neurotransmitter—a chemical released by neurons, or nerve cells, to send signals to other neurons. It helps regulate movement in our bodies. It also regulates pleasure and is released into the brain when we expect or receive a reward.

When you shake someone's hand, pat them on the back, and communicate with them, it increases your and their dopamine levels. Dopamine also increases when you accomplish a task, when you laugh, and even when you eat vegetables. If you are feeling down, just love on somebody, or focus on how much God loves you. When you reach out to others and help them feel better, and when you reach out to others to ask them for support, you will increase your dopamine. Doing either requires a decision. Remember, God equipped us to make choices for ourselves.

The role of dopamine in our bodies shows a direct correlation among the spirit, mind, and body. When we study God's Word, pray, sing hymns, or praise Him, it increases our dopamine levels. That makes us feel better emotionally, and then we will feel better physically.

When we experience something pleasant, the release of dopamine makes us want to experience that feeling of pleasure again. That's one reason why drug use often leads to addiction. When people use drugs like nicotine, heroin, or cocaine, it increases their dopamine levels and momentarily makes them feel great. That rush prompts them to continue using drugs, even though they are extremely harmful.

The better way to deal with life's stressors is the God prescription. Acknowledge Him. Ask Him for help, and seek His wisdom as you address the stressors in your life. Then believe and act on what He asks you to do. Your dopamine levels will increase as you commune with God. This act of obedience and faith in God will bring calm to you through trusting Him, which will lower your blood pressure. The act of serving others, His current prescription for sowing seed, will also decrease your blood pressure.

A love relationship increases dopamine, just as food or a drug does. When you are communing with the Lord and you have an insatiable desire to spend time with Him and His people, it is a good addiction. God has set us up to win because dopamine reinforces good habits and breaks down the negative loops. Dopamine will override bad memories. His Word is literally medicine to us.

Replacing Traumatic Memories with God's Love

> You were raised from death with Christ. So live for what is in heaven, where Christ is sitting at the right hand of God. Think only about what is up there, not what is here on earth. Your old self has died, and your new life is kept with Christ in God. Yes, Christ is now your life, and when he comes again, you will share in his glory (Col. 3:1–4, ERV).

Every event we experience is processed and stored in our brain structures. The mind and body can readily access these memories, which will lead to either a positive or negative phys-ical and emotional response. These events ultimately lead to edifying or destructive behaviors, which in turn lead to gain or loss.

Here is an example of one way that memories can affect us neg-atively. We remember the good feelings that "comfort food" gave us as children. If we experience emotional trauma as an adult, we might eat the same comfort foods to activate a cas-cade effect that leads to comfort. If you are feeling stress from life's pressures, you might eat a bag of potato chips because one of your happy childhood memories is of eating potato chips and sandwiches while picnicking in the park with your fam-ily. Eating chips drowns out the stress by increasing dopamine and retrieving or recreating comforting childhood memories of good, protected times when you ate potato chips. Similarly, many of us associate the smell of popcorn with the pleasurable experience of seeing a great movie. But eating high-fat, high-salt foods in excess can lead to increased salt intake, weight gain, and high blood pressure.

A positive version of this scenario is that, when you seek com-fort from emotional trauma, you instead focus on God's Word to comfort you.

This is so powerful! Instead of eating away discomfort, you be-come empowered by the Holy Spirit to renew your mind. That leads to positive emotional and physical cascades and culmi-nates in an improved quality of mental and physical life. You gain peace that surpasses all understanding. You can find this peace only in Christ.

To disrupt the negative cycle of trauma leading to illness, spend time and focus on God's love. This is necessary before we can reach transformational levels of love for ourselves and others.

Love promotes power in our thinking and a sound mind. Love overthrows fear. God gives us the ultimate example of how to overcome fear and anxiety. He acted by thinking of others first. As a brain surgeon in practice for almost twenty years who has treated tens of thousands of patients, I can tell you what love and fear look like.

We know how this works. We know what accomplishments and goal achieving feels like long after the achievement has passed. This gives us hope for a bright future.

> I have loved you as the Father has loved me. Now continue in my love. I have obeyed my Father's commands, and he continues to love me. In the same way, if you obey my commands, I will continue to love you. I have told you these things so that you can have the true happiness that I have. I want you to be completely happy. This is what I command you: Love each other as I have loved you. The greatest love people can show is to die for their friends. You are my friends if you do what I tell you to do. I no longer call you servants, because servants don't know what their master is doing. But now I call you friends, because I have told you everything that my Father told me. You did not choose me. I chose you. And I gave you this work: to go and produce fruit—fruit that will last. Then the Father will give you anything you ask for in my name. This is my command: Love each other (John 15:19–17, ERV).

The God Prescription: Strategies to Stop the Loop of Negativity

1. Meditate on the Word of God—the Bible—day and night. This renews your mind and is the answer to all issues related to the soul (mind, will, emotions). There is no other fix for the negative loop of memories that bombard our brains.

2. Focus on how much God loves you. Focus on how much other people love you. Connect with other people to increase your dopamine level. Reach out to others to help them feel better and to ask them for support.

3. If you are a parent, take your children to church, beginning when they are very young. Let them be exposed to Christ's love, the love and acceptance of others who love God, the power of prayer, and the Word of God. This will equip your children with the best possible strategy for coping with life's disappointments and tragedies.

6

Worrying Damages Us Spiritually, Mentally, and Physically

Do not be anxious or worried about anything, but in everything [every circumstance and situation] by prayer and petition with thanksgiving, continue to make your [specific] requests known to God. And the peace of God [that peace which reassures the heart, that peace] which transcends all understanding, [that peace which] stands guard over your hearts and your minds in Christ Jesus [is yours] (Phil. 4:6–7, AMP).

Our bodies cannot sustain prolonged worry. Instead of allowing worries to take control of our minds and throw us into a state of stress and panic, we can choose to rest on God's love and peace. We must believe that God loves us and wants us to be worry-free and stress-free every day of our lives.

When we worry about things that are beyond our control, that worry continues to be processed in a loop in our minds and memories. Although we can't see or feel that negative loop being processed, it has negative consequences for our health. For example, if your father died prematurely twenty years ago, and you have been worried since then that you will die when you get to be the age he was when he died, that negative thought process can manifest as physical ailments—illnesses—in your body.

In her book *Battlefield of the Mind*, Joyce Meyer says, "Our minds are battlefields because our enemy, Satan, has waged war on us." He is carrying out a strategy to deceive us and fill our minds with worry, doubt, confusion, depression, anger, and feelings of self-condemnation.

These negative emotions and thoughts cause us to doubt the promises God has made so clearly in His Word. That, in turn, can cause us to accomplish less than we are capable of and even to make poor life choices. It often takes a conscious effort to stop worrying and instead start believing God's promises.

Here is Joyce's advice to us:

> Satan wants you to think that you are mentally deficient—that something is wrong with you. But the truth is, you just need to begin disciplining your mind. Don't let it run all over town, doing whatever it pleases. Begin today to "keep your foot," to keep your mind on what you're doing. You will need to practice for a while. Breaking old habits and forming new ones always takes time, but it is worth it in the end.[60]

In our culture, many people have the misconception that you're not a good parent unless you worry about your kids. But worrying doesn't help them or you. Instead of worrying, take positive steps to ensure your children's well-being. Teach

---

60. Joyce Meyer, *Battlefield of the Mind: Winning the Battle in Your Mind* (New York: Warner Books, Inc.), 90.

them how to make wise choices and to avoid danger. Talk with them about their concerns and let them know you love and support them. Those positive steps are far more beneficial than worrying.

We were never meant to handle worry or fear. Don't take it on. It will present itself to you every day, but you don't have to let it in. You are going to be tempted to worry about something 24/7. Be aware when worry creeps into your consciousness, and combat it by repeating God's Word—for example, tell yourself, "Do not worry about tomorrow."

> So do not worry about tomorrow; for tomorrow will worry about itself. Each day has enough trouble of its own (Matt. 6:34, AMP).

How Worry Can Cause Illness

God equipped our minds and bodies with complex mechanisms to process both positive and negative thoughts and experiences.

The physical mechanism called *homeostasis* is the tendency toward a relatively stable equilibrium between interdependent elements, especially as maintained by physiological processes. This mechanism occurs naturally in our bodies, and it can be altered based on what we think. When we focus on negative thoughts and worry, it can lead to chronic stress, which can cause a negative cascade in our physical and mental health. But when we read God's Word, pray, and praise God, we create a positive state of mind filled with joy and well-being.

Then the prefrontal lobe of the brain, which is the lobe that enables reasoning, will send signals to the *hypothalamus*, which is a master gland in the brain. It controls most bodily functions through the nervous system and endocrine system. What happens there has an effect on all the body's organs.

The *cortex* of the brain is the outer layer of the cerebrum (the cerebral cortex). It plays an important role in consciousness. When we worry, the cortex sends signals to the thalamus and hypothalamus and to the rest of the limbic system, which controls emotions. Then a signal is sent to the circuit of Papez, which controls memory.

When you remember a time that was distressing and resulted in a negative outcome, either for you or someone else, you pull that information from your memory banks. Those memories become active information that validates your worry. The same process happens when you hear information that triggers you to worry. From there, the sympathetic and parasympathetic systems are activated. Your nervous system reacts, so your heart rate increases, and you secrete hormones like cortisol that give you the "fight or flight" response. God built these mechanism into our bodies to enable us to handle life- threatening situations.

At this point, you release a massive amount of cortisol, your muscle strength increases, and the flow of blood to your muscles and the rest of your body increases. Your blood vessels become narrower so that blood can get blood shunted to your lungs, legs, heart, and brain, which enables you to run or fight to defeat your foe. But if that negative state continues for too long, then, eventually, you will have too much lactic acid buildup in your muscles.

Over time, your heart becomes worn down. Your autoimmune system is activated, and that leads to a host of other negative results. That physical loop of brain structures, the circuit of Papez, continues.

There is a memory loop that Keith Moore refers to in his podcast from his 2015 series "Careful for Nothing." These loops occur together. The physical loop is the processor of information that our five senses present to us. The loop in our minds, which is spiritual, takes over after this information is processed through the physical loop. These thoughts, which are separate from the brain structures, can stay with you for eternity if you so choose because you are a being that transcends the life span of your body. These are properties of the real you. So if you worry, you don't stop worrying when you go to sleep. While we are sleeping, our brains are still working, just as our hearts are still beating.

Caroline Leaf's geodesic theory explains that the subconscious mind processes at a rate of 400 billion actions per second! A lot goes on at the subconscious level that we aren't even aware of. Two of Dr. Leaf's books, *Who Switched Off My Brain* and *The Perfect You*, highlight these principles and describe these phenomena in detail.

When you wake up, the worry continues in the background, even though you are engaging in work and all your other normal activities. The only way to shut down the negative thought process is to think about something that is more powerful than those thoughts.

People who never address their stress and worry have these negative thoughts running in the background throughout their lives. This leads to physical manifestations, ranging from stomach ulcers to cancer and from autoimmune disorders to psychological disorders. There is a breakdown of the brain and the body. Our five senses become overwhelmed with the negative consequences.

Only God is powerful enough to transcend the negativity that bombards us every day, moment by moment.

In her book *Think and Eat Yourself Smart*, Dr. Caroline Leaf provides this practical, helpful advice: "Do not go to sleep worrying about your circumstances; this can upset your sleep cycle, digestion, and weight. Hand all your issues over to God, and fall asleep quoting a Scripture or thinking of all the good things that have happened to you or anything that makes you happy and feel at peace. Write your cares down before you sleep, and read the promises in God's Word. Give Him your fears."[61]

> Give all your worries to him, because he cares for you
> (1 Peter 5:7, ERV).

Worrying can cause a scenario that we can call "cells gone wild." This process can begin at an early age. If a four-year-old child experiences real trauma (domestic violence in the home) or perceived trauma, he can misinterpret things he can't understand or deal with. Those memories become embedded in his subconscious and play in his mind throughout his life. There is a direct correlation between exposure to unresolved stress in

---

61. Caroline Leaf, PhD, *Think and Eat Yourself Smart: A Neuroscientific Approach to a Sharper Mind and Healthier Life* (Grand Rapids, Michigan: Baker Books, 2016), 232.

a child's life and chronic pain, stress, and fear carried into his or her adult life.

The brain's frontal lobe (the reasoning center) does not fully mature until the age of twenty-five or twenty-six. Therefore, any information or experience that a child encounters will create a chain of thoughts and emotions without any perspective or boundaries at all. The traumatic events could seem minor to an adult with a fully developed frontal lobe. Things that hurt children more than parents realize include horror films, verbal abuse or disrespect from Mom or Dad, and tensions and arguments between Mom and Dad. These are the kind of events that create uncertainty in a child's heart. They go on to develop deep-seated fears that manifest as neurotic or compulsive behavior. Children seek stability, often overcompensating for a lack of it with attempts to control their environment and then realizing it's impossible to control every aspect.

Therefore, what children and young adults see or hear before the age of twenty-six affects their emotional and mental states profoundly. These events generate unusual dreams and memories connected to thoughts that become destructive in their brains and then into their minds.

Let's say you had an uncle who was a smoker, developed lung cancer, and died. You remember that he used to talk about his horrific chest pains. Then one day, you feel a chest pain. You remember your uncle's report of his experience. The memory loops through your circuit of Papez over and over and over, and you become extremely worried that now you have lung cancer, like your uncle. The background for your worry was instability created in you before you found out about your uncle's diagnosis.

This worrying leads to an increase in cortisol and the breakdown of your immune system, which can lead to pathologic disease states— including cancer. Instead of worrying about the chest pain, go to your doctor to find out what is causing it. It could be something simple. If it isn't, wait until you get a diagnosis, and don't worry about which treatment to undergo. Don't assume that a diagnosis is a death sentence.

Remain calm, and focus on all the times when you were injured or sick and were healed. This is the Lord's intention for all His children. Focus on all the people you know and those mentioned in the Bible who were healed because of their faith in God and because of their prayers and the prayers of others that were answered. Then read about the cases of people who were diagnosed with supposedly incurable diseases who were healed, and science can't explain why.

When you focus on those positive thoughts and outcomes, they flow through your circuit of Papez, and then you will have joy in your heart. Your immune system becomes stronger. Your natural killer cells and T-cells, which are usually weak in certain cancers such as lymphoma, are strengthened. Those cells attack cancer cells. All the genes and mechanisms that are the "garbage men" in our bodies will clean up the cancer cells that have replicated. Now your cancerous tumors begin to shrink exponentially.

Because of the stem cells in our bodies, regeneration of tissue occurs when we think about good things. Those positive thoughts will overpower and transcend any physical reality and will have a great impact on our souls and bodies.

God's Word contains only Good News when you are qualified to receive His promises. Meditate on God's Word, and repeat Bible verses when you begin to worry.

> Therefore I tell you, stop being worried or anxious (perpetually uneasy, distracted) about your life, as to what you will eat or what you will drink; nor about your body, as to what you will wear. Is life not more than food, and the body more than clothing? (Matt. 6:25, AMP).

Fear Is One Cause of Worry

> But now, this is what the Lord, your Creator says, O Jacob, and He who formed you, O Israel, "Do not fear, for I have redeemed you [from captivity]; I have called you by name; you are Mine!" (Isa. 43:1, AMP).

Like worry, fear is a damaging emotion, and a learned one. Studies show that we are not born with fear. A baby will not show fear, even if you put her in front of a lion that could eat her, or if you put her at the edge of a cliff where she could plummet to her doom. It means nothing to her. We all come to this Earth without fear, as God would have it.

Fear is a learned behavior, and I believe we learn fear from those we are closest to.

For example, a little boy might pick up a poisonous snake he sees outside and say, "Oh, look at the pretty snake." He has no knowledge of the danger he is in. He has no fear in his heart, so there is no response from his limbic system, and his circuit of Papez is completely quiet. He is calm. There will be no increased cortisol surges that could lead to problems down the road. But then let's say the boy's mother comes along and sees her son holding the snake. She jumps back and screams in fear. The boy senses her fear, so he echoes her scream in a delayed reaction. Now the boy has learned that he should fear snakes.

Most parents are not aware that their children learn to be fearful from them. Being aware that children learn from their parents and model their behavior can lead us to be more thoughtful about our reactions. These are teaching moments. A better reaction is to explain to the child calmly that some snakes are poisonous and can hurt him. Teach him about the different types of snakes. Ask him to move quickly away from any snakes he sees and to alert an adult. Ask him if he has any questions, and answer them in a calm, honest, straightforward way.

Fortify yourself with God's peace surrounding you, and show your children, by example, how to react to bad news, dangerous circumstances, and potential problems in a calm, hopeful, positive manner. Just as we can teach children how to fear, we also can teach them how to cope with life's challenges in a thoughtful manner. We must show our children God's Word so they can experience God's peace for themselves.

God Can Halt the Cycle of Worry

The wonderful news is that God can totally disrupt the entire process of worrying.

When we praise Him, our bodies respond in a positive way. For example, if I am feeling excited, happy, or joyful, my blood pressure will increase, and my heart will pump blood more quickly. Why? Because the hypothalamus communicates through the sympathetic system, which in turn communicates through the sympathetic chain to my heart and blood vessels.

It also helps to add regular exercise, laughing, and thinking about God's wonderful, powerful promises to this process. Faith without effort is dead. Doing so allows us to feel joy, which is a good kind of stress that helps nourish our organs, including our brains and hearts. The result is that we feel a sense of well-being, not only because that feeling of joy activates the sympathetic system, but also because our hormones are activated.

When I am joyful, my body secretes certain chemicals—the good hormones: cortisol, along with growth hormone and the hormones that regulate my sugar level. So now, my sugar level doesn't get out of control because growth hormone is controlling my pancreas, and so forth.

In His infinite wisdom, God built those regulatory mechanisms into our bodies to react to our mental state. When we think on good things, those mechanisms are automatically triggered to benefit us. What we see, taste, hear, feel, and think—every aspect of our physical beings—is transcended when we think about God, His love for us, and what He has done for us, as chronicled in His Bible that we read daily. Jesus's name is above every other name.

When we read God's Word, we see the way God states how things should be. Focusing on our victory over death because of His ultimate sacrifice will enable us to transcend our worries because they are usually of a physical nature. Most of our worries are related to an event's physical consequence, such as receiving a medical diagnosis or learning that a child was injured in an accident. Or death. Jesus took the keys of death. So even death has lost its sting. The transition of dying will feel to us as though we're moving to another place because He took the pain, sting, and anguish out of death. He took punishment for our sins onto His own body, brain, and mind so that we don't have to carry the burden—*if* we believe what Jesus did for us.

When we pray, praise God, and read His Word, we help heal our brains. The pleasure centers of our brains get pleasure from those activities. The same thing happens when we give instead of taking. We get a rush of cortisol.

God says He will never forsake us or leave us. Likewise, He will never forsake or leave our children.

> For He has said, "I will never [under any circumstances] desert you [nor give you up nor leave you without support, nor will I in any degree leave you helpless], nor will I forsake *or* let you down *or* relax My hold on you [assuredly not]!
>
> (Heb. 13:5, AMP).

God also says that if two or more are present and agree on any one thing, then He is faithful and just to answer our prayers.

> For where two or three are gathered in My name [meeting together as My followers], I am there among them (Matt. 18:20, AMP).

Claim that promise. Pray with your spouse or someone else for your child's healing and for your own healing. God's omnipotence supersedes any physical illness or injury that can come your way.

Worry is a natural reaction when we hear bad news. Again, as Joyce Meyer states, "We have to focus on breaking the bad habit of worry."

If you receive a potentially serious diagnosis, focus on God's promises, not on the worst outcome possible. Think and say something like, "God's Word says it, and therefore I say that I am healed. My cells are healed. My liver is healed. My brain is healed. I call my kidneys healed. All the cells in my body are healed and are functioning as they were intended to function without malfunction. I am strong and healthy." Avoid saying or thinking, "I am not in this condition" because that means you are focusing on the bad condition. Think about and meditate only on God's promises.

> Therefore we do not become discouraged [spiritless, disappointed, or afraid]. Though our outer self is [progressively] wasting away, yet our inner self is being [progressively] renewed day by day
>
> (2 Corin. 4:16, AMP).

God's peace will encircle your soul (mind, will, and emotions) and brain when you yield to Him. His peace will be active in your life.

> Therefore, my fellow believers, whom I love and long for, my delight and crown [my wreath of victory], in this way stand firm in the Lord, my beloved
>
> (Phil. 1:1, AMP).

God's aim is to heal our bodies and minds. Our job is to pray and thank God for His miracles and grace, think about His mercy, and stay in faith. Satan delights when our spirits and minds are filled with fear, so he does everything he can to keep us fearful. He wants God's peace to be ineffective in our lives.

> This is your right as royalty. For you have not received a spirit of slavery leading again to fear [of God's judgment], but you have received the Spirit of adoption as sons [the Spirit producing sonship] by which we [joyfully] cry, "Abba! Father!" (Rom. 8:15, AMP).

> There is no fear in love [dread does not exist]. But perfect (complete, full-grown) love drives out fear, because fear involves [the expectation of divine] punishment, so the one who is afraid [of God's judgment] is not perfected in love [has not grown into a sufficient understanding of God's love]

> (1 John 4:18, AMP).

Parables Make God's Teachings Easy to Understand

It is difficult to think about something good if we don't understand it. That's why, in the Bible, God created life lessons in the form of parables, or stories. In this way, God has made the concepts of salvation, forgiveness, and hope easy to understand and memorable so we can benefit the most from them. If we understand those lessons, we can apply them to our own lives in tangible ways. All we have to do is believe Him and claim the victory.

> But my God shall supply all your need according to his riches in glory by Christ Jesus (Phil. 4:19, KJV).

The key is to believe what His Word says over what we see, hear, feel, and think. Believing His Word in the face of any challenging situation will create change. So if you have been diagnosed with cancer, focus on God's Word and message of healing, not the illness. We have to truly believe He has healed us. Often, we do not fully surrender to that belief.

Bruce H. Lipton, PhD, is a former medical school professor and research scientist. In his best-selling book *The Biology of Belief*, he examines in great detail the mechanisms by which cells receive and process information. Lipton concludes that genes and DNA do not control our biology; rather, DNA is controlled by signals coming from *outside* the cells, including the energetic messages emanating from our positive and negative thoughts. His research indicates that our bodies can be changed as we retrain our thinking.

Lipton says, "Your beliefs act like filters on a camera, changing how you see the world. And your biology adapts to those beliefs. When we truly recognize that our beliefs are that powerful, we hold the key to freedom. While we cannot readily change the codes of our genetic blueprints, we can change our minds and, in the process, switch the blueprints used to express our genetic potential."[62]

---

62. Bruce H. Lipton, PhD, *The Biology of Belief: Unleashing the Power of Consciousness, Matter, and Miracles* (Carlsbad, California: Hay House, 2005), 137.

Jesus Implores Us to Understand Spiritual Things

In Matthew 13, we find the "parable of the sower," also called the "parable of the soils." Jesus tells the crowds gathered around him a parable about a farmer who was trying to plant some seed. Jesus explains that some of the seed fell onto the road, and birds ate it. More seed fell on rocky ground without much soil. Plants grew quickly, but because their roots weren't deep, they were scorched by the sun. But some of the seed fell onto good soil and yielded grain. At that point, Jesus's disciples asked Him why He spoke to the people in parables. Here is Jesus's reply:

> Jesus replied to them, "To you it has been granted to know the mysteries of the kingdom of heaven, but to them it has not been granted. For whoever has [spiritual wisdom because he is receptive to God's word], to him *more* will be given, and he will be richly *and* abundantly supplied; but whoever does not have [spiritual wisdom because he has devalued God's word], even what he has will be taken away from him. This is the reason I speak to the crowds in parables: because while [having the power of] seeing they do not see, and while [having the power of] hearing they do not hear, nor do they understand *and* grasp [spiritual things]" (Matt. 13:11–13, AMP).

Jesus goes on to warn people that when they fail to understand what He is trying to teach them (reject God's Word), they open the door for Satan to steal from them the promise of God's Word.

In Matthew 13:19–23, Jesus explains how scenarios with the farmer's seed relate to our spiritual lives, specifically to our hearts. The *wayside* ground is a heart that doesn't believe God's Word. The *stony* ground is a heart that receives God's Word gladly but has no roots in that heart, so any challenge or difficulty will make the Word of no effect. The *thorny* ground is a heart in which the cares of this world choke out the promises of the Word (by the person's choice). *Good* ground is a heart in which the teaching of God's Word is deep in the heart and mind and will easily be chosen over any competing thoughts and will prevail, even in difficult times.

We see this when a person who is full of the Word is soaked in joy because he prefers what Jesus says about his challenging circumstance over how he perceives the circumstance with his senses or heart. Jesus will always allow us to triumph over our challenges:

> When anyone hears the word of the kingdom [regarding salvation] and does not understand *and* grasp it, the evil one comes and snatches away what was sown in his heart. This is the one on whom seed was sown beside the road. The one on whom seed was sown on rocky ground, this is the one who hears the word and at once welcomes it with joy; yet he has no [substantial] root in himself, but is only temporary, and when pressure or persecution comes because of the word, immediately he stumbles *and* falls away [abandoning the One who is the source of salvation]. And the one on whom seed was sown among thorns, this is the one who hears the word, but the worries *and* distractions of the world and the deceitfulness [the superficial

pleasures and delight] of riches choke the word, and it yields no fruit. And the one on whom seed was sown on the good soil, this is the one who hears the word and understands *and* grasps it; he indeed bears fruit and yields, some a hundred times [as much as was sown], some sixty [times as much], and some thirty (Matt. 13:19–23, AMP).

When we turn our focus from God's promises and choose instead to worry and think negative thoughts, those thought patterns have psychological, emotional, and physical ramifications. If you are upset all the time, it will affect you and others around you negatively, and you will age prematurely. But this is not God's fault. He offers us peace derived from His perfect Spirit; all we have to do is accept it.

He wants us to model our behavior after Him:

The things which you have learned and received and heard and seen in me, practice these things [in daily life], and the God [who is the source] of peace *and* well-being will be with you (Phil. 4:9, AMP).

You Are What You Think About

One of my central messages is that what you think about has an effect on you. This concept is supported in the Bible, too.

For as he thinks in his heart, so is he [in behavior—one who manipulates]. He says to you, "Eat and drink," Yet his heart is not with you [but it is begrudging the cost] (Prov. 23:7, AMP).

Therefore, it's important to focus on things that are good and on solutions, and it's important to have hope. A lot of this hope comes out of the Bible, which is a highly credible piece of literary work. More than any other book from antiquity, the Bible has withstood the most rigorous scrutiny. So, whether someone believes the Bible or not, or is a Christian or not, the Bible offers a significant amount of emotional and spiritual comfort.

A happy heart is good medicine *and* a joyful mind causes healing, but a broken spirit dries up the bones (Prov. 17:22, AMP).

Leland Ryken, PhD, a professor of English emeritus at Wheaton College in Wheaton, Illinois, says the Bible is the world's most famous literary work. He writes, "In fact, it is the central book of English-speaking cultures throughout the ages. It has provided the cohesive frame of reference (what some literary scholars would call the mythological universe) for England and America. Compared to the Bible, even the collected works of Shakespeare are demonstrably in the second tier." Ryken describes the Bible as being in the format of a literary anthology—a collection of varied literary genres written by multiple authors over the span of many centuries...embodied in the genres of narrative, poetry, letters, and visionary writing. Dozens of smaller genres accumulate under those big rubrics."[63]

Some of my acquaintances are atheists. I am not judging them. I don't believe anyone is less of a person because he or

---

63. Leland Ryken, "The Bible as Literature," *The Washington Times*, December 11, 2014, https://www.washingtontimes.com/news/2014/dec/11/ the-bibles-influence-the-bible-as- literature/.

she doesn't subscribe to my views or my faith. God loves His whole creation. They will list reasons why God doesn't exist, and often, their reasons are related solely to the experiences of other people. They will argue, "I know this Christian who is a bad person. Therefore, God doesn't exist." Or they will ask why God doesn't fix a problem or cure an illness. These are not scientific scenarios, yet some of these people are scientists. They will tell you that science does not prove God's existence. They are basing their conclusion on certain data only. There are significant data and natural observations that confirm His presence.

For example, gravity exists, whether or not you believe in it. Likewise, God's existence is not dependent on belief in Him. An argument regarding gravity disproved Stephen Hawking's theory. All-natural phenomena exist or occur because an intelligent being, our Heavenly Father, created them. The so-called "Big Bang" occurred when God commanded, "Let there be light!" Likewise, some do not understand who they are as spirit beings. They are like those who enjoy the benefits of having a brain while never seeing it.

Embracing Our True Spiritual Nature

> Study to shew thyself approved unto God, a workman that needeth not to be ashamed, rightly dividing the word of truth (2 Tim. 2:15, KJV).

We must rightly divide the Word of God, which means we must have good Bible teaching and guidance from the Holy Spirit to interpret the Scriptures accurately. Otherwise, we can create fictitious definitions and wrong interpretations of what God is saying to us in His Word, and we'll have no consistent or accurate guide for our lives. We will become lost without the dependability of God's Word. We are spirits that possess souls (mind, will, and emotions) and live in physical bodies. Bishop Keith A. Butler, my pastor, is a stickler for rightly dividing the Word of God. He has reiterated this correct definition and interrelationship of who we truly are hundreds of times.

If you understand that we are more than just our physical bodies, then at least you will look in the right place for solutions to some of the greatest challenges that civilization, medicine, and science face as they relate to the emotional manifestation of disease processes. The social destruction that we are now seeing, as groups fight each other, is a marker of human hearts that don't grasp their value or God's love for them. Our physical health is partly a reflection of how well we handle stress, what we deem important in our lives, and how we *act* on what we deem important. We must always remember that God loves us and promises to take care of us.

> Consider the ravens, for they neither sow [seed] nor reap [the crop]; they have no storehouse or barn, and yet God feeds them. How much more valuable are you than the birds! And which of you by worrying can add one hour to his life's span? So if you are not even able to do a very little thing [such as that], why are you worried about the rest? (Luke 12:24–26, AMP).

The God Prescription: Strategies to Stop Worrying

1. Give God glory all the time. This will crush fear and uncertainty.

2. Keep Scripture before your eyes at all times. Repeat a Bible verse four times in a row—for example, "Tomorrow will worry about itself."

3. Pray in the Spirit.

4. Remember a time when God helped you solve a serious problem or get through a difficult situation. Think about how hopeful and happy you felt. Focus on that feeling, and place your hope in Him. Find Scriptures that relate to your situation. Place Bible verses in areas where you can see them easily. Believe that He will heal your spirit, mind, and body.

5. Focus on staying relaxed to break the chronic "fight or flight" response. As Keith Moore says, God's thoughts are not nothing, nor are our thoughts nothing. God's Word, the Bible, contains His thoughts, regardless of what language the words are written in. His thoughts are the same. They have power and can become your thoughts as you choose to accept them. His thoughts are life-giving and will replace negative thoughts because they are so powerful.

6. Read psalms and listen to spiritual songs that penetrate your heart so that God can transform your negative thinking and worry into hope and peace.

7. Earnestly keep faith in God during tough times. Believe that He will deliver you from your situation.

8. Choose not to be upset or overly concerned about anything.

> So for the sake of Christ, I am well pleased and take pleasure in infirmities, insults, hardships,

persecutions, perplexities and distresses; for when I am weak [in human strength], then am I[truly] strong (able, powerful in divine strength) (2 Corin. 12:10, AMPC).

9. Cast down any thought that is placed above God's thoughts.

Casting down imaginations, and every high thing that exalteth itself against the knowledge of God, and bringing into captivity every thought to the obedience of Christ; and having in a readiness to revenge all disobedience, when your obedience is fulfilled

(2 Corin. 10:5–6).

7

How Laughter Can Help Heal

Blessed [joyful, nourished by God's goodness] are you who hunger now [for righteousness, actively seeking right standing with God], for you will be [completely] satisfied. Blessed [forgiven, refreshed by God's grace] are you who weep now [over your sins and repent], for you will laugh [when the burden of sin is lifted]

(Luke 6:21, AMP).

The best source of laughter is overflowing joy that comes from an intimate relationship with Jesus Christ. The only way to establish this relationship is by accepting Jesus Christ as your personal Lord and Savior. This means that you say with your mouth and believe in your heart, "I believe that Jesus Christ is the Son of God and that He died on the cross for my sins. I ask forgiveness and confess my sins to You, Lord. You rose on the third day after going to hell in my place. You, Jesus, are now seated at the right hand of God, and because of what You did for me, I am born again."

Laughter is good medicine. It regulates your immune system in a way that protects your body against disease and minimizes its destructive effects.

And Sarah said, God hath made me to laugh, so that all that hear will laugh with me (Gen. 21:6, KJV).

Patch Adams: A Pioneer in Laughter Therapy

If you saw the movie *Patch Adams,* starring Robin Williams, you know who Hunter "Patch" Adams is. Hunter Doherty "Patch" Adams, MD, is an American physician, comedian, social activist, clown, and author. Dr. Adams treats children and others with major illness by applying the benefit of laughter. His was the first nonpartisan, private-sector effort to address cancer and other terminal disease states with an emphasis on the soul (mind, will, and emotions), and body (brain).[64]

In 1971, Dr. Adams founded the Gesundheit! Institute. The basis for this nonprofit health-care organization is a paper he wrote that encouraged the medical community to focus on "whole systems thinking" and to integrate that type of thinking with the hospital–community concepts that emerged in medical school. Dr. Adams describes the Institute as "a project in holistic medical care based on the belief that one cannot separate the health of the individual from the health of the family, the community, the society, and the world." His mission is to reframe and reclaim the concept of "hospital."[65]

---

64. Patch Adams website, http://www.patchadams.org/global-outreach/faqs/.
65. Ibid.

An interesting aspect of Dr. Adams's work is his "clown trips." In 1985, he took a group of people on a clown trip to what was then the Soviet Union. Equipped with colorful clothing and compassion, the group visited hospitals, orphanages, and homes for the elderly. Now those trips are an integral part of Gesundheit's global outreach. He and his team visit war zones, refugee camps, and natural-disaster sites. They have built clinics and a school at some of the places they have visited. Dr. Adams goes on six or seven of these trips yearly.[66]

I applaud Dr. Adams's pioneering and innovative work that looks at wellness through a lens entirely different from that of most physicians.

TIME Magazine's Special Edition on Laughter

In 2018, *TIME* published a special edition of its magazine titled "The Science of Laughter: Our Bodies. Our Minds. Our Souls." The collection of articles presents an account of how ancient philosophers like Aristotle appreciated wit and humor. It also explains that laughter is an important communication tool, as well as a natural remedy for many different ailments.

The authors write, "Recent research has lauded laughter as a remedy for arthritis, backaches, Alzheimer's, itching, allergies, heart disease, muscle cramping, and of course, stress. Laughter may boost immune function, pain tolerance, cardiovascular health, and memory." The article also mentions several

---

66. Ibid.

indications that laughter is increasingly helping people manage health issues:[67]

- A university hospital in Pittsburgh runs a twenty-four-hour television station devoted to humor.

- There is a Health and Humor Association in North Carolina.

- Several hospitals affiliated with the University of California, Las Vegas, sponsor the much-celebrated "Rx Laughter," a program that integrates funny movies while administering difficult medical treatments, such as chemotherapy and dialysis.

Simply by laughing, we can release stress. Your body doesn't recognize the difference between a spontaneous laugh and a laugh you emit on purpose, just to feel better. All kinds of laughter are beneficial, thanks to our loving God!

MD Anderson Cancer Uses Laugh Yoga as a Treatment

In fact, laughter is such good medicine that the world-renowned MD Anderson Center uses laughter yoga to facilitate the healing of cancer patients. According to the center's website, "We all know that laughter makes us feel good. Laughter fills your lungs and body with oxygen, exercising your lungs.

---

67. "The Science of Laughter: Our Bodies. Our Minds. Our Souls," *TIME Magazine Special Edition*, June 28, 2018.

Participants report reduction in stress, blood pressure, depression, and more."[68]

William Baun, the Wellness Officer at MD Anderson Cancer Center, hosts laughter yoga classes for cancer patients and caregivers. Here is what he says about the positive effects of laughter:

> Research shows stress weakens our immune systems, can cause body resistance to treatments, and disturbs the healing process. Laughter is a positive sensation that balances the chemical and hormones of the body. It triggers the release of endorphins, the brain's own painkiller, and promotes an overall sense of well-being. Laughter yoga is group exercise for the nervous and cardiovascular systems and our spirits. It's a mix of clapping, chants, laughter, and child playfulness. The good news is that your body can't differentiate between real and fake laughter, so the mantra in laughter yoga classes is "fake it till you make it."[69]

The Fascinating Science Behind Laughter

The physiological study of laughter has its own name: "gelotology." Research has shown that laughing is more than just a person's voice and movement. Laughter requires the coordination

68. "Laughter Yoga," MD Anderson Cancer Center events page, http://www3.mdanderson.org/calendar/event/Laughter_Yoga_9750.html.

69. "Laughter Yoga, MD Anderson Cancer Center," LinkedIn, March 19, 2015, https://www.linkedin.com/pulse/laughter-yoga-md-anderson-cancer-center-william- baun-epd-cwp-fawhp.

of many muscles throughout the body. Laughter is beneficial to us because it can do the following:

1. Increase blood pressure (momentarily, like exercising)

2. Increase heart rate (momentarily, like exercising)

3. Change breathing

4. Reduce levels of certain neurochemicals (catecholamines, hormones)

5. Boost the immune system

6. Aid in relaxing by reducing muscle tension

Laughter is good medicine. When you are feeling sad, despondent, or depressed, make yourself laugh. Again, your body doesn't know whether you are laughing spontaneously or are forcing yourself to laugh. The benefit is the same either way!

There are some cases in which a good, deep laugh might help people with respiratory problems by clearing mucus and aiding in ventilation. Perhaps laughing can also help cardiac patients by giving the heart a bit of a workout. Some hospitals even have their own "Humor Rooms," "Comedy Carts," and clown kids in attempts to speed patients' recovery and boost morale.

How laughter affects the nervous system and rest of the body is not completely understood. A new area of neuroscience called *psychoneuroimmunology* studies the interactions between the brain and the immune system. The field of psychoneuroimmunology combines the methods and techniques of psychology, neuroscience, and immunology. Psychoneuroimmunological experiments usually focus on how stress affects the nervous system and disease states.

Laughter has been shown to cause changes in the autonomic nervous system and to alter stress hormone and neurotransmitter levels. For example, in one study, watching a sixty- minute video of the comedian Gallagher caused reductions in the levels of cortisol, growth hormone, and catecholamines.

A paper published in the journal *Nature* titled "Electric Current Stimulates Laughter" provides more information about how the brain is involved with laughter.[70]

The paper discusses the case of a sixteen-year-old girl, "A. K." who was having surgery to control seizures due to epilepsy. During surgery, the doctors electrically stimulated A. K.'s cerebral cortex to map her brain. Brain mapping is done to determine the function of different brain areas and ensure that brain tissue to be removed is not serving an important function.

The doctors noticed that A. K. laughed whenever they stimulated a small (2 cm by 2 cm) area on her left superior frontal gyrus (part of the brain's frontal lobe). This area is part of the supplementary motor area. Unlike laughter that happens after brain damage, the laughter that was produced in A. K. by electrical stimulation also had a sense of "merriment or mirth." Also, A. K. did *not* have the type of epilepsy with gelastic seizures. Each time her brain was stimulated, A. K. laughed and said that something was funny. The thing that she said that caused her to laugh was different each time. A. K. laughed first and then made up a story that was funny to her. This was unusual because most people first know what is funny, and then they laugh.

---

70. I. Fried, C. L. Wilson, K. A. MacDonald, and E. J. Behnke, "Electric Current Stimulates Laughter," *Nature 391*, no. 650, 1998.

The authors of the paper believe that the area of the brain that caused laughter in A. K. is part of a larger circuit involving several different brain areas. Different parts of the circuit may be important for the following:

1. The emotions produced by a funny situation (the emotional aspect of humor)

2. The "getting it" part of a joke (the cognitive, thinking aspect of humor)

3. Moving the muscles of the face to smile (the motor aspect of humor)

Other areas of the brain, such as the temporal lobe and hypothalamus, may also participate in laughter and humor.

Laughing Related to Tickling

So now we know a little more about what part of the brain is responsible for humor. But this doesn't explain why we laugh or why we don't laugh when we tickle ourselves. Believe it or not, there has been some research in this area. In fact, researchers at the University of California in San Diego have even constructed a "Tickle Machine." For these scientists, tickling is no laughing matter!

Some scientists believe that laughing caused by tickling is a built-in reflex because even babies do it. If this is true, then you should be able to tickle yourself...but you can't, can you? Even if you try to tickle yourself in exactly the same way another person tickles you, you don't laugh. Why? The information sent to your spinal cord and brain should be exactly the same. Apparently, for tickling to make you laugh, the brain needs tension and surprise. When you tickle yourself, you know exactly what will happen; there is no tension or surprise. How the brain uses this information about tension and surprise is still a mystery, but there is some evidence that the cerebellum might be involved.

Everyone smiles and laughs. It is possible that smiling, laughing, and tickling are used to create bonds between babies and parents. When a parent tickles a baby and the baby responds with a smile or laugh, the parent laughs and smiles, too. In this way, the baby and parent get to know one another, and the baby learns all about laughter by watching and responding to a parent. What a happy way to learn!

Further research into how a positive attitude affects a person's health need to be done. This will give a whole new meaning to the phrase "fun science."

> Then our mouth was filled with laughter and our tongue with joyful shouting; then they said among the nations, "The Lord has done great things for them"

> (Ps. 126:2, AMP).

The God Prescription: Strategies to Activate God's Mechanisms to Heal Yourself with Laughter

1. Laugh, even when you don't feel like it.

2. Watch or listen to some shows by comedians who do not use obscenities, like Carol Burnett, whose Emmy-winning variety show, *The Carol Burnett Show*, aired on CBS from 1967 to 1978. A Christian comedian who is popular today is Tim Hawkins.

3. Read comics in the newspaper or comic books.

4. Watch funny videos on YouTube, such as the eT-rade babies or videos showing the hilarious antics of children and animals.

8

Stem Cells:
The Origin of Life and
the Mechanism for
Healing

*Before I formed you in the womb I knew you [and
approved of you as My chosen instrument], And before
you were born I consecrated you [to Myself as My own];
I have appointed you as a prophet to the nations*

(Jer. 1:5, AMP).

One night, I was reading my daughter a bedtime story. While we were sitting in her bed talking, she said," Daddy, didn't God make Eve from Adam's rib?"

I said, "Yes honey."

The next thing I thought about was the pluripotent stem cells I study and on which I seek the Lord's direction. The Holy Spirit said to me, "Eve was made from the stem cells in Adam's rib." I picked myself up off the floor after receiving this major revelation, and then I gave the Lord praise for allowing me to have this information.

So the Lord God caused a deep sleep to fall upon Adam; and while he slept, He took one of his ribs and closed up the flesh at that place. And the rib which the Lord God had taken from the man He made (fashioned, formed) into a woman, and He brought her *and* presented her to the man. Then Adam said, 'This is now bone of my bones, and flesh of my flesh; she shall be called Woman, because she was taken out of Man. For this reason a man shall leave his father and his mother, and shall be joined to his wife; and they shall become one flesh (Gen. 2:21–24, AMP).

Adam's rib contained bone marrow, which stores stem cells. I believe God used those stem cells to create Eve. We have seen how adult stem cells derived from bone marrow have been used to make and reproduce tissues and organs. So it makes sense that our Creator created Eve using the same technique that He uses to heal us.

God put an immune system in us with "soldier" cells that kill cancer cells, infections, and other disease processes. An everyday instance that demonstrates the Lord's love for us physiologically is how quickly we heal after we cut our skin.

A scab forms, which is a complex fibrin lattice that allows the stem cells and other tissue to fill in the gap in the skin tissue. When the scab falls off, we see new skin without any trace of injury. Now, surgeons assist by cutting away dead cells and disinfecting wounds when intervention is needed. However, the surgeon doesn't heal the patient: he or she helps patients heal through the work that God performed when He formed us.

Faith Activates Healing

> Pleasant words are as an honeycomb, sweet to the soul,
> and health to the bones (Prov. 16:24, KJV).

People who are ill are often healed only seconds or minutes after faith is activated or ignited when faithful followers of Christ lay hands on them or when the Lord deposits His Word into their spirits. Because stem cells are regenerative, our injuries can be healed.

This phenomenon creates a cascade of events through an epigenetic phenomenon of DNA and brain-matter changes that cause communication between certain brain centers and our bone marrow and immune system. That leads to a super-charged activation of stem cells, which then leads to the gradual (or rapid) production of cells needed to help heal us. This healing happens when damaged tissue or a malfunctioning organ is repaired.

Your faith activates this complex God-engineered process that could repair any severely damaged limb or organ. I know that this seems wild, but it is explainable with an understanding of stem-cell purpose and function as a backdrop. The "switch" that activates or accelerates this process is our faith that we are healed by His grace from that moment onward.

Of course, life is sometimes difficult. It is reasonable to be perplexed—but not in despair. If we are upset, nervous, or depressed, it's because we do not trust God and what He said. This is a heart problem, not an intellectual/head/mental/cognitive problem.

When you have faith in God, it doesn't mean you are denying the problem or challenge you face. It means you act wisely with the information presented to you and seek His guidance. Again, you have to make a *choice*. The way people handle hardship reveals their level of spiritual maturity.

You can abide in God's peace and withstand the storms of life. Keep your peace, love, and joy as you navigate life's challenges. He will be with you, every step of the way. What a powerful witness of God's goodness working in us!

> He who dwells in the shelter of the Most High will remain secure *and* rest in the shadow of the Almighty [whose power no enemy can withstand]. I will say of the Lor d, "He is my refuge and my fortress, my God, in whom I trust [with great confidence, and on whom I rely]!" (Ps. 91:1–2, AMP).

As a neurosurgeon, I perform a type of spine surgery in which I have to remove a portion of a rib to gain access to the spine. Before I conduct this surgery, I explain to the patient and family during the consultation visit that I will have to remove a portion of one or two ribs. I emphasize that it is safe. I assure the patient that he or she will not have any substantial pain or negative repercussions from this technique. The patients who have this procedure usually do well. They don't miss the portion of rib that I removed! God performed this surgery after He put Adam to sleep, long before we ever used this same technique. It sounds barbaric, but it is not. It works!

God Knew Us Before We Were Born

God created us with stem cells, which make us grow from two physical cells—the sperm and the egg—to trillions of cells over time. He put stem cells and complex mechanisms in our bodies just for the purpose of repair and continued health!

An intelligent being had to create that process: evolution will not explain it. Although Darwin had some amazing observations, and there is a place for evolution, it does not explain how human life began. The theory of evolution has been so wildly taken out of proportion that it makes no sense anymore.

We are not just a bunch of molecules put together by random events and an evolutionary process, as secularists might believe. We are fearfully and wonderfully made. We were knit together in our mothers' wombs from the moment of conception, when thirty-four chromosomes become forty-six.

> For You formed my innermost parts; You knit me [together] in my mother's womb (Ps. 139:13, AMP).

Scripture is scientific, yet God uses examples we can understand. He gives us simple instructions to follow.

Stem cells make other cells, and they can be repaired. When you have an incision or cut in your skin, blood clots form from fibrin to stop the bleeding. Eventually, stem cells replace that huge gash to the point where it's a thin scar, and you have normal tissue. And you completely forget that it even happened to you. That is part of the healing mechanism God built into our incredibly complex bodies.

The immune system is also a part of that same complex system. God knew we would be at risk of infection and disease processes, so He equipped us with a very strong immune system that kills intruders. Our immune systems came from stem cells, as did the rest of our bodies. Again, we grew from two cells to trillions of cells. Our hair, nails, and skin are constantly regenerating. The platelets in our blood regenerate. Even our palates—our taste buds—regenerate. All these reparative mechanisms happen because He created them.

Stem Cells Have the Potential to Treat Diseases

Recent studies have shown that neural stem cells (NSCs) are present in the subventricular zone (SVZ) that lines the lateral ventricles and the subgranular zone (SGZ) of the hippocampal dentate gyrus (DG) in adult mouse, rat, nonhuman primate, and human brains. A 2007 study revealed that newly generated cells in the SGZ can differentiate into mature, functional neurons and integrate into the DG as granule cells, which are involved in memory formation. This means it might be possible for damaged cells to be replaced from endogenous neural stem cell pools. The researchers concluded that we could use pharmaceutical tools to manipulate the proliferation, migration, and neuronal differentiation of endogenous NSCs to reach the adequate benefits for the treatment of central nervous system diseases.[71]

---

71. Jin K and Galvan V., "Endogenous Neural Stem Cells in the Adult Brain," *Journal of Neuroimmune Pharmacology 2*, no. 3 (September 2007): 236–42, https://www.ncbi.nlm.nih.gov/pubmed/18040856.

Brains Continue Making Cells, Even in the Elderly

In April 2018, researchers at Columbia University presented new evidence that our brains continue to make hundreds of new neurons a day, even after we reach our seventies, in a process known as *neurogenesis*.

Researchers examined the brains of twenty- eight healthy people ranging in age from fourteen to seventy-nine who had died suddenly of accidents but not long-term disease. They found that "older people made as many new neurons in parts of the brain responsible for memory as younger people do." However, the aging brains had reduced blood flow to nourish these cells. In other words, "the pool of new brain cells is still there, but it's not as active in older brains," the study revealed.[72]

Plasma Can Restore Damaged Joints

Regenerative orthopedics, or RO, is a nonsurgical approach whereby physicians use small, precise injections of platelet-rich plasma, or PRP, with or without stem cells to regenerate damaged joints, ligaments, and tendons. PRP is rich in the body's own growth factors and is spun down from a simple blood draw that takes about half an hour.

Stem cells are typically harvested from a patient's own abdominal fat in a simple office-based surgical procedure. The doctor then processes the fat to yield the stem-cell injectate, which

---

72. Deborah Netburn, "Surprise! Scientists Find Signs of New Brain Cells in Adults as Old as 79," *Los Angeles Times*, April 5, 2018, http://www.latimes.com/science/ sciencenow/la-sci-sn-new-brain-cells-20180405-story.html.

takes a couple of hours. Then the doctor injects the PRP at the precise location of injury or degeneration and stimulates the body to "regenerate" the damaged structure. These injections are safe and can yield impressive results with many orthopedic and musculoskeletal conditions.[73]

That is another example of how God created our bodies to heal.

Epigenetics: How Changes in Gene Expression Can Affect Our Health

Epigenetics is the study of changes in organisms caused by modification of gene expression—not by alteration of the genetic code itself. It falls in with the spirit–soul–body connection from the standpoint that we have genes, but not all genes are expressed automatically. They are often altered by outside forces such as diet, exercise, and negative or positive emotions.

Stem cells have been a focus in neurosurgery for spinal cord injury to brain tumor formation to bone/spine fusion using stem-cell transplant. Likewise, immune system and brain tumors, as well as infection treatments, have been discussed for years around these reactions and exchanges occurring in the brain. Epigenetics helps us understand how we have regeneration and replacement of the hippocampus in the brain and memory function.

Emotions are directly connected to and regulate immune/hormonal events on an epigenetic/cellular level, causing physical and psychological changes to an individual's brain wiring and body. One example of this phenomenon is that a person can

---

73. Joseph Christiano, ND, *Living Beyond Your Chronic Pain: Simple Steps to a Pain-Free and Healthy Life* (Destiny Image Publishers, Inc., 2014).

develop a gastrointestinal ulcer simply by thinking about a negative event that has happened or might occur.

The question often arises whether a medical condition is the result of genetics or environment—the classic "nature vs. nurture" discussion. Dr. Caroline Leaf, an accomplished neuroscientist, explains epigenetics this way:

> Essentially, people, plants, animals, and other living organisms start with a certain genetic code—the "nature" part of the well- known nature/nurture concept—at conception. Yet the choice of which genes are "expressed," or activated, is strongly affected by influences in terms of epigenetics. These environmental influences are the "nurture" part of the equation: the social, emotional, cultural, and economic environments we grow up in.
>
> God has set up a beautiful interplay between us, our biology, and our environments. Due to this exchange, the expression of genes can change rapidly over time: genes are influenced by internal and external factors, and those changes can be passed along to our offspring."[74]

Exercise Promotes Physical Healing

Regular exercise builds new cells in the hippocampus, which plays a role in short- and long-term memory. Studies have shown that aerobic workouts can stave off age-related mental decline and help with recovery from traumatic brain injuries.

---

74. Caroline Leaf, PhD, *Think and Eat Yourself Smart*, 145.

Wendy A. Suzuki, PhD, is an expert in the physiological benefits of exercise. She is a professor of neural science and psychology in the Center for Neural Science at New York University. At a TEDWomen 2017 conference, she said that after gaining twenty-five pounds, she began to exercise. She noticed that the endorphins from her workouts were improving her mood and giving her more energy. She also maintained focus better and read reports more easily.

So she began researching how exercise affected her own lab results and discovered the incredible positive effects exercise has on people's brains and health. She says the prefrontal cortex and hippocampus are the two areas of the brain that are the most susceptible to neurodegenerative diseases and normal cognitive decline in aging. Suzuki says that the more you work out, the bigger and stronger those two areas of the brain become.

Through Suzuki's startup, Brain Thrive, she hopes to give people exercise "prescriptions"—detailed instructions for when to work out, how long, and what to do. The instructions will be tailored to each individual, based on his or her unique health concerns.[75]

Suzuki's research is great news for all of us. Here is an excerpt from her talk:

> Exercise is the most transformative thing you can do
> for your brain today. It has an immediate effect on

75. Hilary Brueck, "A Neuroscientist Is Trying to Create Tailored 'Exercise Prescriptions' for Aging to Keep the Brain Sharp," *Business Insider,* December 4, 2017, http:// www.businessinsider.com/neuroscientist-wendy-suzuki-exercise-prescription-cell-phone-2017-12.

your brain. A single workout will immediately increase levels of neurotransmitters like dopamine, serotonin, and noradrenaline. A single workout can improve your ability to shift and focus attention, which will last for two hours. A single workout can increase your reaction time.

With increased exercise over your lifetime, you're not going to cure dementia or Alzheimer's disease, but you are going to create the strongest, biggest prefrontal cortex and hippocampus so it takes longer for these diseases to take effect. Bringing exercise into your life will not only give you a healthier life today; it will also protect your brain from incurable diseases and change the trajectory of your life for the better. [76]

To get the optimum benefit from exercise, Suzuki recommends getting at least thirty minutes of aerobic exercise three or four times a week. You should exercise hard enough to get your heart rate up.

Exercise is a *choice*. God equipped us with the ability to benefit from exercise, but every day, we must choose to activate our God-given restorative abilities by spending time moving our bodies.

The God Prescription: Strategies to Help Heal Your Physical Body

1. Take care of your body—it is a temple of Christ.

76. Wendy Suzuki, PhD, "The Brain-Changing Effects of Exercise," TED Talk, November 2017, https://www.facebook.com/TED/videos/10160545401360652/.

2. Get at least thirty minutes of aerobic exercise three or four times a week. Exercise hard enough to get your heart rate up.

3. Actively engage your faith to promote healing. Pray, have believers lay hands on you and lay hands on yourself, study His Word, and praise Him aloud.

4. Believe God for everything. Keep calm when you face life's challenges, and stay in faith regarding His intent for you. Abide in faith.

Therefore humble yourselves under the mighty hand of God [set aside self-righteous pride], so that He may exalt you [to a place of honor in His service] at the appropriate time, casting all your cares [all your anxieties, all your worries, and all your concerns, once and for all] on Him, for He cares about you [with deepest affection, and watches over you very carefully] (1 Peter 5:6–7, AMP).

What good is it, my brothers and sisters, if someone claims to have faith but has no deeds? Can such faith save them? Suppose a brother or a sister is without clothes and daily food. If one of you says to them, 'Go in peace; keep warm and well fed,' but does nothing about their physical needs, what good is it? In the same way, faith by itself, if it is not accompanied by action, is dead (James 2:14–17, KJV).

I will give thanks *and* praise the Lor d, with all my heart; I will tell aloud all Your wonders *and* marvelous deeds. I will rejoice and exult in you; I will sing praise to Your name, O Most High…The Lor d also will be a refuge *and* a stronghold for the oppressed, A refuge in times of trouble; And those who know Your name [who have experienced Your precious mercy] will put their confident trust in You, For You, O Lor d, have not abandoned those who seek You (Ps. 9:1–2, 9–10, KJV).

Who against hope believed in hope, that he might become the father of many nations, according to that which was spoken, so shall thy seed be. And being not weak in faith, he considered not his own body now dead, when he was about an hundred years old, neither yet the deadness of Sarah's womb: He staggered not at the promise of God through unbelief; but was strong in faith, giving glory to God; And being fully persuaded that, what he had promised, he was able also to perform. And therefore, it was imputed to him for righteousness (Rom. 4:18–22, KJV).

Now it was not written for his sake alone, that it was imputed to him; But for us also, to whom it shall be imputed, if we believe on him that raised up Jesus our Lord from the dead (Rom. 4:23–24, KJV).

Peace I leave with you, My [own] peace I now give and bequeath to you. Not as the world gives do I give to you. Do not let your hearts be troubled, neither let them be afraid. [Stop allowing yourselves to be agitated and disturbed; and do not permit yourselves to be fearful and intimidated and cowardly and unsettled (John 14:27, KJV).

9

"The Spark of Life"

BASICS

I had an elderly clinic patient who presented with leg pain and back pain. While I was creating a plan of care for her complaints, she mentioned that she had a foot ulcer that had been treated at a wound care clinic for 2 years with no improvement. Given the fact that most people are way behind in their nutritional intake, I suggested that she try an organic powdered food supplement called *Cardio Miracle®* that I had recently learned about and was taking. I knew that there were some great health-promoting ingredients contained in it. It turns out that my hunch was correct. This patient's non healing foot ulcer healed to a pin hole size in just over 2 months of doing nothing different but adding the Cardio Miracle food to her diet!!

You can't tell me that when our bodies are depleted of so many good nutrients that it doesn't become difficult to heal. We go on to have nutritional deficiencies that eventually lead to immunity and regenerative system breakdown and malfunction.

Unfortunately, I wasn't taught much in medical school about nutrition. In fact, education in nutrition was virtually nonexistent. We had 1 segment of a biochemistry class focused on metabolism and nutritional science. The emphasis was largely placed on pharmacological remedies. I believe that there is clearly a place for both, but the emphasis needs to be on supporting the natural healing mechanisms that God has placed in us.

I can't help but think of how many ailments that aren't completely addressed by my current recommendations, that could be addressed with optimizing good nutritional food consumption first.

As a neurosurgeon, I have seen poor wound healing and protracted infection treatment courses largely due to the lack of help from my patients' innate regenerative systems. How can I expect good wound healing after surgery in people with poor nutrition? I can't!

We try to give them more protein intravenously and orally in different settings. However, do we think any further about the specific components of a nutritionally rich diet that supports gut, liver, brain, and bone health? The answer again is that, in general, we don't.

I have learned to be a bit more critical after these last several years. Basic root cause analysis and shared decision making with my patients regarding the risks and benefits of nutrition optimization, conservative care, and procedural intervention is appropriate for the best patient outcomes.

Nitric oxide and its metabolism holds almost a supernatural place in physical and emotional health, as molecular biologists, like Judy Mikovits, maintains.

CARDIO MIRACLE

What is Cardio Miracle?

At a Holistic Medicine conference in 2023, John Hewlett handed me a packet of powder that I mixed into a bottle of water to drink while he shared his story with me. I discovered that he had narrowly survived complications from a routine appendectomy that exacerbated his heart problems. When the doctors recommended a quadruple bypass surgery, he knew that it was time to find a better solution.

This brush with death launched Hewlett on a quest to discover natural and effective ways of improving his cardiovascular and overall health. His quest eventually led him to nitric oxide and the formulation of a supplement that contains the best ingredients for promoting the natural production of nitric oxide in the body: Cardio Miracle.

Cardio Miracle is the complete nitric oxide solution. It is a fine blend of over 58 natural ingredients, including organic beets, carrots, coconut water, cherries, blueberries, spinach, broccoli, pomegranates, grapes, combined with the best amino acids, such as arginine and citrulline. These ingredients work together synergistically to promote and sustain the body's natural production of nitric oxide. Hewlett and his team decided to call the product "Cardio Miracle" because the miracle of God's physical healing power is enhanced inside the body when it produces nitric oxide at optimal levels.

More than 20 years of research and over 100,000 clinical studies have established nitric oxide as a "miracle molecule." Cardio Miracle is unique because of its proprietary dual-pathway nitric oxide delivery and the cellular benefits that have been clinically validated at the University of Ohio in the laboratory of Professor Tadeusz Malinski. Cardio Miracle is also unique because of its therapeutic vitamin D3 delivery, organic fruits and vegetables, inflammation fighting formula, low glycemic index, natural sweeteners, low calories, and high nutrients. It is the supplement to replace most other supplements. That's a big part of why I started taking and recommending it to my patients.

The University of Florida Medical Research Group called nitric oxide, "The spark of life in the cell."

10

What is Nitric Oxide?

This chapter relays more detail on the history and benefits of nitric oxide, including the discoveries and work of Dr. Louis J. Ignarro, and other researchers, and the history and benefits of nitric oxide and the nutrients that developed into Cardio Miracle. My purpose is to persuade every reader to experience for himself or herself the benefits that John Hewlett and many others, including myself, have experienced from daily good food intake with Cardio Miracle.

THE HISTORY

The following is a succinct timeline into the discovery and evolution of learning about nitric oxide:

1869: Alfred Nobel revolutionizes the world by stabilizing nitroglycerin to create dynamite. His factory workers, suffering from angina, discover that handling nitroglycerin alleviates their chest pain. Nobel's own doctor would later prescribe nitroglycerin for Nobel's heart disease, marking the beginning of a remarkable journey in cardiovascular health.

1980: Robert F. Furchgott makes a groundbreaking discovery of an unknown molecule that signals vascular muscle cells to relax. He named this molecule EDRF (Endothelium-Derived

Relaxing Factor), setting the stage for a new era in medical science.

1986: Dr. Louis Ignarro, with relentless determination, proves through a series of analyses that EDRF is identical to nitric oxide. This revelation propels the scientific community into a frenzy of excitement and innovation.

1998: Robert F. Furchgott, Ferid Murad, and Dr. Louis Ignarro are awarded the 1998 Nobel Prize in Physiology or Medicine for their revolutionary discovery "concerning nitric oxide as the signaling molecule for the cardiovascular system." This accolade is a testament to their unwavering perseverance and dedication.

2000: The dawn of a new millennium sees many companies and scientists passionately working to create L-arginine based supplements to boost natural nitric oxide. Some succeed more than others, but the race for excellence is on!

Nitric oxide, or NO, is a short-lived gas produced in the wall of arteries and veins. Its production is signaled by amino acids or other ingredients. Nitric oxide is the body's most powerful natural antioxidant. There are over 100,000 medical studies now validating its importance and beneficial impact on cellular health. As mentioned above, the Nobel Prize in Physiology or Medicine was awarded in 1998 for the role of nitric oxide in reversing heart disease and other cardiovascular problems.

Why do you need nitric oxide?

Nitric oxide supports the immune system, repairs the vessels of the body, fights inflammation, delivers vital nutrients to the cell, and helps facilitate the exchange of oxygen and carbon dioxide. It relaxes arteries and repairs their lining (endothelial cells), and as a mega-antioxidant, even breaks down biofilms that lead to chronic illness and disease.

The Cardio Miracle Formula

John Hewlett's odyssey to create the Cardio Miracle formula began with his early consultations with Dr. Joseph Prendergast and Mike Rosales whose nitric oxide formula (Pro Argi 9) with Synergy Worldwide turned his health around in 2007 and 2008. Over the next six years, Hewlett met with Dr. Siva Arunasalam of the High Desert Heart Institute, who recommended several improvements to the Prendergast formula. Hewlett also held a heart symposium which included Dr. Rainer Boger from Germany, one of the preeminent experts on arginine resistance, who had some research on ingredients, and Dr. Robert Young, expert in PH alkalinity and author of the worldwide bestselling book The PH Miracle.

In 2012, Hewlett met with Dr. Dean Friesan to work on several formula ideas. Dr. Friesan, a doctor of pharmacy, debated and discussed many ideas and concepts about ingredients that were valuable in the delivery of nitric oxide, combatting free radicals, and increasing absorbability. As an important part of his education on the topic, Hewlett spent many hours with Dr. Friesan discussing amino acids and other aspects of nitric oxide delivery. Together they formulated Cardio Flow. Cardio Flow was a precursor to Cardio Miracle that exposed Hewlett to the many challenges associated with ingredients, manufacturing, and supplement formulation in general. Later, nitric oxide supplementation preserved Dr. Friesan's life after he experienced nearly complete heart failure, and even a heart transplant.

During John Hewlett's five years marketing work with Synergy International, he extolled the miracle of his own recovery through nitric oxide therapy, and he devoted his full attention to his new career path. He immersed himself in the science, as he endeavored to share this therapy with the world. He constantly inquired and suggested improvements to Synergy's flagship product, Pro Argi 9 plus. Early in the process, Hewlett informed the other leaders of Synergy that it would be necessary to find an alternative to sucralose, especially for customers who were more health-conscious. It was a major battle. Ph.D.'s and other managers argued for the cost-savings and taste benefits of sucralose versus organic stevia as a sweetener. Hewlett finally prevailed, and the company reluctantly introduced a stevia alternative. Within six months the stevia version of the product was outselling the sucralose version by a ratio of 4 to 1!

Hewlett's next battle against corporate opposition arose when he suggested that the company offer multiple canisters of thirty servings at a bundled price. Hewlett prevailed once again, and a three-pack was introduced with lower commissions and manufacturer suggested retail pricing. Within months this offer became the top-seller in the line.

Hewlett's final battle at Synergy began when he recommended a product for health professionals that would build the credibility of the science and expand the markets. After management reviewed it, the recommendation reached the highest level of Nature's Sunshine Products, the parent company and 350-million-dollar pioneer in the multi-level-marketing industry. Hewlett met with the CEO. The CEO considered that Hewlett's idea for marketing to medical professionals wouldn't work in multi-level marketing because of the high margins that it required. Exasperated, Hewlett determined that it would soon be time to leave Synergy even though he was earning more than a million dollars annually as one of the top distributors.

Hewlett had fought for and helped to fund the patient study with Dr. Arunasalem and his surgical nurse Dan Austin, and he wanted Synergy to retain and fund additional clinical work with Dr. Siva. Management revisited the idea, but they were afraid that the product might not achieve the desired outcome. **They refused to believe that which Hewlett had observed with thousands of customers, namely, that solid scientific studies produce great results. Flabbergasted and frustrated, Hewlett decided to walk away from Synergy sixty days later.** He walked away from what could have been a lifetime, six-figure annuity for his six years of effort.

In the fall of 2013, Hewlett met with a nutritional Ph.D. who helped him to find a manufacturer for the newly created Cardio Miracle formula. Hewlett tested the samples, improved the flavor, and collaborated with manufacturers, including a Ph.D. chemist who coordinated the new samples. But Hewlett was concerned about quality controls. After flying to Atlanta to investigate the manufacturer, Hewlett terminated the consultant, the manufacturer, and future orders in order to search for a facility of higher quality.

He finally found a manufacturer in Southern Utah. One of the major benefits of the new manufacturer was to meet Robert Dickman, the senior Vice President of product development.

Over the next several years John Hewlett and Robert Dickman spent hundreds of hours together testing ingredients, flavors, and different formulations in the effort to improve Cardio Miracle. After consulting with Dickman, Hewlett learned that, in most instances, active ingredients of high quality are as good as the more widely known trademark brand names that require millions of dollars in research and advertising.

Hewlett taught Dickman about much of the nitric oxide science, including the benefits of nitric oxide in combating free-radical damage. From early on, Dickman was amazed by Hewlett's commitment to quality. Dickman had been used to dealing with formulations that were driven primarily by profits, and not by results. But Hewlett spared no expense in his efforts to develop the finest possible product that would achieve the best possible results for customers.

Over the next four years, Hewlett collaborated at length with the manufacturers and chemists who provided many good ideas about active ingredients and helped to educate him in many ways. **Hewlett and his team spared no expense in proving the best of the best in quality ingredients and effective nitric oxide delivery. Whereas many supplement companies develop their products merely in order to generate the biggest financial profits, John Hewlett cut no corners with the Cardio Miracle formula.**

In the spring of 2019, Hewlett met with Tadeusz Malinski Ph.D, the premier scientist on Vitamin D3 and nitric oxide testing at the cellular level. Malinski and his workers in his University of Ohio laboratory tested the Cardio Miracle formula for its delivery at the endothelial level. The astonishing results were published in February 2020. Hewlett's efforts over a 13-year educational process were finally validated. It was gratifying to confirm the benefits of the Cardio Miracle formula in the laboratory of a renowned scientist. **To the best of Hewlett's knowledge, there has never been testing of a nitric oxide supplement at this level anywhere else in the world.**

What I find very assuring as a supplement, is that Cardio Miracle contains **no artificial colors, no GMO's, no synthetic ingredients, and no inexpensive fillers.** It contains a **unique blend of amino acids, vitamins, minerals, and antioxidants that support its proprietary dual-pathway nitric oxide delivery, through the sublingual pathway and the gut.** This means that release of nitric oxide begins when it is even swished around in the mouth before swallowing and then further creation of NO when absorbed through digestion. It is formulated to support nitric oxide levels for an extended period, while supporting anti-inflammatory protection with 5000mg of antioxidants.

One of the **key ingredients** in the Cardio Miracle formula is grape seed extract. **Grape seeds and grape seed extract have a wide variety of health benefits ranging from cardiovascular health to cognitive function.** Grape seed extract can benefit any diet by helping the body to naturally produce nitric oxide. It also works as a particularly strong antioxidant. It contains protein, carbohydrates, and fats, but it also contains a category of antioxidants called polyphenols. Scientific studies have shown that **grape seeds have fifty times more antioxidant power than vitamin C.** Grape seed extract also benefits collagen, the bones, and the brain.

For the best results, the recommended intake of Cardio Miracle is twice daily, spaced twelve hours apart, morning and evening. It is best to avoid taking Cardio Miracle within thirty minutes of any protein in order to allow maximum absorption and effectiveness. One of the great things about Cardio Miracle is that it tastes good, and for me, that makes it easier not to forget if it is enjoyable. **It is also much more convenient to drink Cardio Miracle than to try to swallow dozens of pills, with dubious capacity for absorption, each day.**

11

The Benefits of Good Food Nutrients from Cardio Miracle

I used to start my morning routine by digging through my pantry cupboard to find the supplements I would regularly take. These included: Turmeric, Vitamin C, Vitamin D3, Vitamin A drops, Quercetin, Elderberry, Zinc, and Black cumin seed. This was especially true during the height of the COVID-19 pandemic. Virtually all of these have been replaced by the morning routine of enjoying a glass of Cardio Miracle, because of the nutrient and antioxidant content in it. A full night's sleep, the elimination of coffee and energy drinks, the reduction or elimination of toxic foods, regular moderate exercise, better hydration, and Cardio Miracle twice a day will greatly contribute to improved energy levels.

It makes sense that improvement in one area of the body can contribute to improvement throughout the body. Enhanced nitric oxide accomplishes this very thing, beginning with the endothelium and progenitor cells. Progenitor cells are repair cells that fill in the rips and tears created by toxins in our blood stream. As we age (specifically as we pass the age of forty) the repair process conducted by progenitor cells slows down because nitric oxide production diminishes significantly. The stimulation of natural nitric oxide production, therefore, can reduce or reverse the obstacles to the work of progenitor cells.

As we age, the endothelium, or blood vessel lining, becomes more rigid. Rigid blood vessels make it more difficult for blood to flow smoothly, which leads to cardiovascular problems, and a potential host of other debilitating problems. Nitric oxide, the production of which is greatly enhanced by Cardio Miracle supplementation, causes the endothelium to relax, to soften, and to become less rigid, which in turn supports healthy blood pressure and eases the burden on your heart. Nitric oxide keeps blood vessels flexible and smooth so that blood can easily reach the vital parts of the body:

- Reduces blood pressure
- Increases blood flow and oxygenation
- Increases vitamin D uptake and efficacy
- Improves cellular health and reproduction
- Improves cardiovascular health
- Prevents blood clotting that causes strokes and heart attacks
- Nourishes the heart, lungs, intestines, blood vessels, white blood cells, lymphatic system, insulin receptors, the olfactory sense, and the brain
- Positively affects the function and well-being of the entire human body
- Resolves erectile dysfunction
- Increases sexual stamina and health

Moreover, nitric oxide benefits overall health and fitness by

- Increasing energy
- Increasing clarity of mind
- Improvement in pain
- Decreasing inflammation
- Stress reduction

These benefits of these nutrients are available almost immediately after ingesting Cardio Miracle for the first time. In fact, it is often advised to swish it around in the mouth before swallowing, because nitric oxide is produced even in this first part of digestion where it is easily absorbed in the oral mucosa, that is, the inside lining of our mouths. More importantly, though, there are long-term benefits to long-term use of Cardio Miracle. In order to explain why Cardio Miracle is so effective and has so many benefits, it is important to consider the detailed scientific support for Cardio Miracle. If you are a science buff, you may thoroughly enjoy pouring over this chapter. If you are not, you may want to breeze over these pages. Either way, I am compelled to lay out my personal exploration on the topic which convinced me as to why I will take this product daily for the rest of my life, and why I can't think of one situation where someone would not benefit from taking it themselves.

Scientific Support for Cardio Miracle:
The Malinski Study

Dr. Tadeusz Malinski's advanced study of nitric oxide contains a detailed scientific description of the benefits of Cardio Miracle. In essence, Malinski's study confirms that nitric oxide is a crucial signaling molecule that regulates blood flow and prevents adhesion of blood components to the vascular wall, and that Cardio Miracle increases the amount and the bio-availability of nitric oxide in the system.

A signaling molecule is a molecule that transmits energy, information, or a state of one cell to another. In order for a signaling molecule such as nitric oxide to be effective, it must also be bioavailable, that is, capable of proper assimilation into the body. A deficiency in bioavailability of nitric oxide may lead to chronic illness or diseases such as diabetes, atherosclerosis, hypertension, and so forth. The deficiency in bioavailability of nitric oxide harms the endothelium of all blood vessels (capillaries, veins, aorta, heart, etc.) which increases oxidative stress and other problems such as clots or the build-up of plaque. Malinski's study proves that Cardio Miracle favorably increases nitric oxide ratios and the bioavailability of nitric oxide as well as the other antioxidants and vitamins. His study also proves that the promotion of optimal levels of nitric oxide in the body helps to relax the blood vessels which leads to a wide variety of improvements for health and fitness.

The methods and technology necessary to complete Malinski's experiments are themselves amazing. Without going into too much detail, Malinski tested healthy human endothelial cells with Cardio Miracle from Evolution Nutraceuticals, and measured ratios of nitric oxide and peroxynitrite (a harmful free radical) by means of small sensors and other ingenious devices. The results of Malinski's experiment were astounding:

He showed that this supplement not only caused immediate nitric oxide production, but that it created the right environment for nitric oxide to be produced in blood vessel lining and initiate healing and improved blood flow.

Incredibly, Malinski's laboratory was the first in the world to measure the production of nitric oxide in a single endothelial cell, in vivo in humans, and in the beating heart. Furthermore, Malinski was able to perform measurements of bioavailable nitric oxide produced by a single endothelial cell in different segments of the cardiovascular system, such as capillary vessels, the aorta, and the heart. These studies clarify concentrations of nitric oxide and peroxynitrite in the presence of elevated concentrations of Vitamin D3, L-arginine, L-citrulline, and several antioxidants (i.e. Cardio Miracle). The composition of Cardio Miracle consists of two major groups: 1. L-arginine, L-citrulline, and Vitamin D3, which can directly influence endothelial(blood vessel inner wall) nitric oxide synthase (eNOS), and 2. antioxidants that reduce the level of oxidative stress.

The Malinski study shows that nitric oxide is a gaseous molecule that is generated by the NOS enzyme, stimulated by calcium flux, and synthesized from L-arginine, a non-essential amino acid, and oxygen. As mentioned previously, nitric oxide has at least two important functions in the cardiovascular system, namely as a crucial signaling molecule that regulates blood flow and as a molecule that prevents adhesion of blood components, cells, or bacteria in the bloodstream. It stimulates smooth muscle relaxation and dilation of the arteries, increasing the velocity and volume of the transportation of blood. It is important to note that the Malinski study also confirms that nitric oxide signaling regulates blood flow in the brain through capillary vessels, and blood flow is vital to long-term memory.

Malinski measured the ratios of nitric oxide (NO) to peroxynitrite (ONOO-), the latter of which, along with superoxide, is a component of oxidative stress. Higher levels of bioavailable nitric oxide reduce oxidative stress, which is a common factor in chronic diseases and problems such as diabetes, stroke, heart attack, neurodegenerative diseases such as Alzheimer's and Parkinson's disease, and aging. Malinski's proven hypothesis is that restoring and maintaining optimal levels of bioavailable nitric oxide reduces levels of oxidative stress, which is helpful in targeting the aforementioned diseases. Simply put, Cardio Miracle enhances the body's natural production of nitric oxide, which in turn makes it easier for the blood to flow and to deliver the nutrients and the nitric oxide that cells need in order to thrive.

The first part of Malinski's study investigates the short-term benefits of Cardio Miracle, and the second part of his study pertains to the long-term benefits of Cardio Miracle. Malinski found that "a mixture of L-arginine, L-citrulline, Vitamin D, and antioxidants significantly increases the concentration of bioavailable cytoprotective (cell-protective) nitric oxide", and that at the same time "the level of cytotoxic (cell-destructive) peroxynitrite (ONOO-) decreased." Thus, the ratio between these two important signaling molecules in endothelial cells improved by about 50%, which is "the bottom line in preserving the function of the cardiovascular system." In other words, Malinski proved that Cardio Miracle promotes the body's natural production of nitric oxide which works to protect, preserve, and improve our cardiovascular system.

Malinski concludes that the benefits of Cardio Miracle are based on two important factors: the L-arginine/nitric oxide pathway and the reduction of oxidative stress. He demonstrates that Cardio Miracle facilitates optimal nitric oxide production and ratios which in turn lead to improvement in cardiovascular health. As many scientists and researchers, including Dr. Ignarro, Dr. John P Cooke, Dr. Stamler, and Dr. Sinatra, have also affirmed, improved cardiovascular health leads to dramatic improvements in overall health and fitness.

The purpose of Malinski's study was to estimate how efficient and beneficial Cardio Miracle could be in the enhancement of the endothelial function and efficiency of the cardiovascular system. Malinski discovered that it is not just the total production of nitric oxide, but the production of bioavailable nitric oxide (or nitric oxide that survives for at least 1 to 6 seconds in the biological environment of our bodies) that is important in the proper function of the cardiovascular system.

Malinski's data clearly indicates that the level of toxic peroxynitrite produced by the endothelium decreased significantly after treatment with Cardio Miracle for up to 12 hours. Therefore, the recommendation of taking Cardio Miracle twice a day (every 12 hours), makes perfect sense; you would potentially maintain the protective effects of nitric oxide production in the blood vessels, while keeping oxidative stressors in the blood at a reduced level. Malinski and his team found that a deficiency in bioavailable nitric oxide and/or an excess of O-, is a common denominator of several diseases such as hypertension, diabetes, stroke, aging, heart attack, and many other neurodegenerative diseases such as Alzheimer's disease, Parkinson's disease, epilepsy, and migraine. Therefore it is crucial for the maintenance of the cardiovascular system to produce biologically optimal levels of nitric oxide and low levels of peroxynitrite. Cardio Miracle greatly facilitates both of these positive results.

Malinski's study also confirms that the long-term treatment of the endothelium with Cardio Miracle improves endothelial function and restores the function of damaged cardiovasculature from the effects of disease. The prevention and treatment of disease requires a restoration and maintenance of high levels of bioavailable nitric oxide and a reduction of oxidative stress. As shown by this study, Cardio Miracle performs both of these functions. Moreover, Cardio Miracle produces optimal concentrations of nitric oxide close to the surface of the membrane (endothelial cell) which is important because the surface concentration of nitric oxide influences nitric oxide diffusion and propagation, which in turn regulates smooth muscle relaxation and the optimal diameter of blood vessels.

The Emergent Studies

Emergent Study 1: "Effect of Cardio Miracle on Vitamin D Efficacy and Atherosclerosis"

Building upon Dr. Malinski's advanced study of nitric oxide and the benefits of Cardio Miracle, Dr. Anton Franz Fliri and his team at Emergent System Analytics have used the proprietary technology Emergent Intelligence (EI) to further delineate Cardio Miracle's mechanisms of action in cardiovascular disease, particularly atherosclerosis, and to investigate its health benefits beyond the cardiovascular system. Thus far they have discovered that Cardio Miracle increases oral availability of cholecalciferol (Vitamin D), increases cellular uptake of calcitriol (the active form of Vitamin D3), and activates cellular processes known to enhance Vitamin D effectiveness. They also discovered that the synergistic interactions between Cardio Miracle ingredients support cellular mechanisms that are known to prevent the development of atherosclerosis and initiate regression of the disease.

Dr. Fliri and his team's unique technology works to discover cause and effect relationships resulting from protein network interactions at a system-wide scale. They describe in detail the more than fifty ingredients in the Cardio Miracle blend, and how these ingredients work together to produce the aforementioned benefits. Every ingredient has been meticulously chosen, but some of the most important ingredients include arginine, citrulline, cholecalciferol, a phytonutrient blend, quercetin, and other minerals and natural products. The combination of arginine and citrulline in the formula is particularly important because it increases arginine levels in the blood that fuel the production of nitric oxide from nitric oxide synthase (NOS). Folate and minerals such as calcium, magnesium, potassium, are also important because they support the activity of nitric oxide synthase (eNOS) along the blood vessel lining (endothelium) and lower cellular peroxide levels; and the addition of Vit D to the formula, some of which is extracted from Shiitake and Maitake mushrooms, also enhances nitric oxide generation.

Quercetin and catechins found in abundance in Cardio Miracle's antioxidants increase the efficacy and oral availability of Vitamin D. This is significant for many reasons, not the least of which is because Vitamin D deficiencies are associated with debilitating conditions such as bone resorption disease, hyperglycemia, CoQ10 deficiency disease, rickets, and osteoporosis.

Dr. Fliri and his team also confirmed that Cardio Miracle supports caveolar functions. Caveolae are small (50-100 nm) cavities in the plasma membranes of many cell types. Caveolae regulate transport across cell membranes and transport cargo enriched with receptors and ion channels (caveolae mediated endocytosis, or CME). Cardio Miracle helps to activate CME. Cardio Miracle's core ingredients work together synergistically to support several molecular functions and a feedback loop that increases nitric oxide production. This support of molecular functions and the feedback loop that increases nitric oxide has been reported to impede progression of atherosclerosis and cause regression of established disease.

Furthermore, **Cardio Miracle activates autophagy**. Autophagy is the body's method for purging damaged cells in order to regenerate fresh, healthy cells. Cardio Miracle activates autophagy through ingredients such as palmitic acid, resveratrol, pterostilbene, quercetin, piceatannol, delphinidin, cyanidin-3-o-glucoside, and sulforaphane. Cardio Miracle's multiple and mutually supporting anti-atherosclerotic mechanisms of action support Cardio Miracle's potential for supporting the treatment of atherosclerosis.

In sum, Dr. Fliri's application of the Emergent Intelligence technology shows that Cardio Miracle not only corrects cellular activity imbalances that cause endothelial dysfunction, but it also enhances the efficacy and bioavailability of Vitamin D.

The molecular mechanism driving Vitamin D efficacy enhancement rests on Cardio Miracle's capacity to increase levels of bioavailable nitric oxide and to inhibit protein kinase C which, in turn, activates and supports transport functions of caveolae. This mechanism of action supports functions of a feedback loop that increases nitric oxide production, increases Vitamin D efficacy, and decreases oxidative stress. In these and other ways, supplementation with Cardio Miracle supports treatment of atherosclerosis and assists treatment of conditions caused by nitric oxide and Vitamin D deficiencies.

Emergent Study 2: "Cardio Miracle for Diabetes"

Building on the previously mentioned studies, Dr. Anton Fliri and the Emergent System Analytics team next studied the effects of Cardio Miracle on biological processes involved in the development and progression of diabetes. They discovered that Cardio Miracle possesses a number of functionalities that are ideally suited for intercepting development and progression of diabetes and associated comorbidities.

This second Emergent study is especially important because current treatments for diabetes that target single mechanisms of action are insufficient. These current treatments are insufficient because they fail to integrate mechanisms of action that support the integrity of insulin receptor signaling, insulin secretion, and healthy pancreatic cell function and renewal. Furthermore, current strategies for the treatment and prevention of diabetes do not adequately protect against microvascular complications that lead to diabetes associated comorbidities.

Sadly, over 1 in 10 people of the U.S. population have type 2 diabetes (T2D), and 1 in 3 are pre-diabetic. More than 30% percent of those with T2D suffer from at least one complication, such as coronary artery diseases, hypertension, dyslipidemia, high LDL cholesterol, neuropathy, retinopathy, nephropathy, and cognitive decline. One of the key risk factors for T2D is chronic inflammation and cardiovascular disease associated with obesity. Thus, causes of diabetes involve overproduction of proinflammatory cytokines triggering inflammatory conditions that damage insulin secreting pancreatic islet β-cells and lead to decreased responsiveness of β-cells to glucagon-like peptide-1 (GLP-1) and glucose-dependent insulinotropic polypeptide (GIP). These problems lead to hyperglycemia. Hyperglycemia, in turn, causes endothelial(inner blood vessel wall) dysfunction. Thus diabetes is not only a metabolic disease but also a cardiovascular disease. In fact, ischemic stroke accounts for most of the morbidity, hospitalizations, and death in patients with diabetes.

How does Cardio Miracle help? In order to understand the positive effects of Cardio Miracle for those who suffer from problems associated with diabetes, it is important to consider how nitric oxide affects the root causes of cardiovascular and metabolic diseases.

During the very early stages of diabetes, there is a loss of insulin release which predicts development of hyperglycemia. These early states called prediabetes are also associated with a pseudo-insulin resistance which alters insulin responses and insulin clearance. More advanced stages of disease progression involve development of insulin resistance, when pancreatic cells become exhausted, which accelerates development of full-blown diabetes and associated comorbidities. A common premise linking obesity, onset of cardiovascular disease and insulin resistance is an imbalanced nitric oxide production. Thus, the **bioavailability of nitric oxide is decreased in cardiovascular disease, obesity, and development of insulin resistance.**

The decline of nitric oxide levels in obesity is, therefore, one of the root causes of problems associated with diabetes. Lower nitric oxide production also harms the caveolae(intake mechanisms) of the cells.

The results of this **second Emergent Study, therefore, are that Cardio Miracle supports eNOS-mediated nitric oxide generation** through the combination of arginine, citrulline, and cholecalciferol Vitamin D, and inhibits iNOS(an enzyme that makes Nitric Oxide from Arginine) -mediated nitric oxide generation through the action of the Cardio Miracle ingredient, quercetin, which is an iNOS inhibitor.

Nitric oxide derived from endothelial(or inner blood vessel wall)NOS (eNOS) activates caveolae-mediated endocytosis which (1) increases insulin receptor sensitivity; (2) prevents pancreatic cell dysfunction and decreases inflammation, (3) reverses impairment of glucose and arginine-stimulated insulin secretion, and (4) decreases excessive transforming growth factor-β receptor signaling, which prevent a harmful feedback loop. The combination of these functionalities allows Cardio Miracle to support pancreatic regeneration and improve the outcome of diabetes and associated comorbidities. Cardio Miracle helps to support the body's repair of root causes of cardiovascular and metabolic disease.

The Frontiers in Nutrition Report

In their article "Functional Characterization of Nutraceuticals Using Spectral Clustering: Centrality of Caveolae-Mediated Endocytosis for Management of Nitric Oxide and Vitamin D Deficiencies and Atherosclerosis," Dr. Anton Franz Fliri and Shama Kajiji elaborate on the scientific support for the benefits of Cardio Miracle. Their main discovery was that Cardio Miracle helps to correct cellular redox imbalance because of its ability to increase oral bioavailability of cholecalciferol vitamin D3 and to activate and stabilize caveolin-mediated endocytosis.

As we've seen from the previous studies, this essentially means that Cardio Miracle stimulates an increase in nitric oxide production, vitamin D3 efficacy, autophagy, and down-regulation of TGF beta activity. These positive effects, in turn, are anticipated to inhibit or reverse the endothelial dysfunction that is one of the root causes of diseases such as atherosclerosis, diabetic kidney disease, and COVID-19. "Supplementation with Cardio Miracle…" Fliri and Kajiji conclude, "is projected to benefit treatment of these diseases," and "clinical trials are warranted" to validate these predictions.

Other Studies

There are many other scientific studies that highlight the benefits of nitric oxide in the body and thus lend support to the efficacy of the Cardio Miracle formula.

In 2006, researchers at the University of Florida conducted a study to determine activities in the body on a molecular level that cause life-threatening problems associated with diabetes and atherosclerosis. They discovered that the problems had to do with cellular responses to vascular injury. The cells in the bodies of diabetic patients did not repair themselves adequately, but when nitric oxide gas was added, the cells became less rigid and began to move about normally. Nitric oxide facilitates the transport of repair cells out of the bone marrow, directing them to the necessary areas for the necessary repairs to the endothelium. Thus, nitric oxide is the key to activating these repair cells.

In 2009, Dr. J. Joseph Prendergast and Dr. Siva Arunasalam of the High Desert Heart Institute, one of the most prestigious heart institutes in the United States, conducted a clinical study of 33 patients who had experienced congestive heart failure, exhausted their pharmacological and medical treatment options, and were left with only one remaining option: a heart transplant. During the 90-day extensive study, each patient received regular diagnostic testing to determine and measure results in as many areas as possible, and the study generated almost 7,000 points of data.

During the study, each patient received 20 grams of L-arginine combined with L-citrulline, vitamin D, and other ingredients that support nitric oxide production and heart health. After the study, Dr. Arunasalam observed that every patient showed tremendous improvement, including "positive remodeling of the heart, positive pulmonary artery changes, pulmonary vascular changes in terms of pulmonary pressures, changes in the cardiac dimensions, changes in heart function," and each one of the 33 patients returned to their normal activities. The heart-transplant candidates no longer required the procedure.

Another study at the Case Western Reserve University Medical Center, published in 2015, led by the aforementioned Dr. Jonathan S. Stamler demonstrated that nitric oxide must accompany hemoglobin to enable blood vessels to open and then supply oxygen to tissues. This study transformed the way that we think about nitric oxide and a healthy respiratory cycle. It proved that nitric oxide inside the red blood cell creates vasodilation, and that the lack of nitric oxide causes severe hypoxia.

There are **over 100,000 other scientific studies on the benefits of nitric oxide,** and the number continues to grow. The field of nitric oxide research is simply inexhaustible. As many doctors, scientists, and researchers have observed, nitric oxide has limitless potential for protecting against disease, positively influencing every organ in the body, and dramatically influencing overall health and fitness in positive ways. Nitric oxide, therefore, is crucial to our health and well-being, and I have found the **Cardio Miracle formula to be the finest supplement I have come across for enhancing the body's natural capacity to produce nitric oxide.**

12

Inspiring Cardio Miracle Testimonials

Now that we've reviewed the history and benefits of nitric oxide and the history and benefits of Cardio Miracle, along with the scientific studies that support them, let's take a look at how these discoveries have blessed the lives of many different individuals in a variety of unique circumstances.

We've already seen how nitric oxide was a crucial component of John Hewlett's own recovery from severe heart problems and iatrogenic harm, and how his research led him to formulate Cardio Miracle. But how has Cardio Miracle blessed the lives of many many others who take it daily?

After his discovery of nitric oxide and his firm resolve that it literally saved his life, John Hewlett walked away from a booming industry and business to begin a new mission to introduce nitric oxide to others who suffer. Everyday Hewlett meets people who suffer from symptoms of joint pain, fatigue, heart problems, stress-related issues, or poor nutrition (often caused by depleted soil from over-farming and the use of pesticides) – all of which are common human afflictions that nitric oxide has been shown to alleviate. When Hewlett began to hear the positive results of Cardio Miracle usage from customers, he also began to understand that his own purpose in life had been revealed to him.

Here are a few true stories of real people whose lives have been positively impacted by Cardio Miracle. These individuals have shared their own "Cardio Miracle".

Avery M Jackson III, MD

Throughout the years as a neurosurgeon, I have stood in the operating room for many hours a day. Some surgeries could last upwards of 12 hours. Leg cramps were not an infrequent end-of-day symptom for me. Hot baths and extra water would help some after the fact, but would never prevent them. After a few months of taking Cardio Miracle regularly, I noticed that I didn't have cramps anymore, even after standing for several hours. That alone convinced me that this was not just another multi-vitamin supplement. That is why I take it every day and have no reservations recommending it for all my patients, family, and friends.

G. Edward Griffin

G. Edward Griffin is a filmmaker, entrepreneur, and author of the excellent book, **The Creature from Jekyll Island**. He has called Cardio Miracle "the most powerful, effective supplement," and a product that has helped him to experience improvements in his health and blood pressure. Griffin had major blood pressure problems before he started taking Cardio Miracle. After supplementing with Cardio Miracle, Griffin stated that he has the "blood pressure of a young man," and that he feels better than he has felt in a long time. Of all the nitric oxide boosters that he has tried, he observed, "Cardio

Miracle is hands-down the most effective". Griffin endorses Cardio Miracle as "the best supplement" that he has ever found.

Scott Palmer

Scott Palmer's friendship with John Hewlett extends over many decades. When Palmer had surgery on his broken leg, Hewlett visited him and introduced him to Cardio Miracle. Palmer's doctor was amazed because he had never seen a scar like his heal so well. Palmer attributes this result in part to daily supplementation with Cardio Miracle. The improvement in blood flow, the reduction in inflammation, and other factors contributed to Palmer's rapid and complete recovery.

Ken Shelton

For John Hewlett's good friend Ken Shelton, Cardio Miracle has been the perfect gift. It did more for him in one year than medicine had done in the previous forty years. The neuropathy in his fingers and toes disappeared. He sleeps better. He is healthier, stronger, and more energetic than ever. Cardio Miracle gave him a sense of health security that he didn't get from the pharmaceutical industry or established medicine.

Scott Proctor

Scott Proctor, Publisher of Meridian Magazine, has struggled with high blood pressure, diabetes, heart disease, low energy, and the challenge of finding the right supplements to alleviate his suffering. He began taking Cardio Miracle, morning and evening, and after 110 days, he got his blood work done. To his delight, everything had improved. His blood pressure that had been high and climbing toward hypertension came down to 120/68. His blood sugar test showed that it was in a range that was just right for him. His good cholesterol that had never been right was finally in a good range. His vitamin D levels were perfect.

Since Proctor hadn't been doing anything else differently except for taking Cardio Miracle, all of these positive benefits pointed to one conclusion: Cardio Miracle supplementation really works. Proctor observed that another bonus of Cardio Miracle is that it is so easy to take. It is simple. A scoop of powder added to water, twice a day, replaces a fist full of hard to swallow pills with vitamins that might never absorb into the cells that need them.

Since supplementing with Cardio Miracle, Proctor has discovered that he has more energy, and that his body has been energized by the influx of nitric oxide. Because he is a fierce advocate of his own health, Proctor has decided to take Cardio Miracle for the rest of his life.

Greg Matsen

Greg Matsen, creator of Cwic Media, has researched natural supplements for a long time. He has filtered through many different kinds of supplements, searching for the best supplements with the most reliable scientific studies to support them. When Hewlett introduced him to Cardio Miracle, Matsen did what he does with all of his work: he began to thoroughly research the sources.

In addition to doing his own research, Matsen wanted to experience Cardio Miracle for himself. He discovered that nitric oxide plays a crucial role in many neuro-biological processes and organ systems in the body. Since he has suffered from kidney problems and other health problems, Matsen has learned how important optimal blood flow is for his own health.

Within approximately thirty days of supplementing with Cardio Miracle, Matsen began to notice particular benefits, for his immune system, his heart health, and his exercise routine. At a fairly young age, Matsen had emergency, open-heart, triple-bypass surgery. Because of this experience, he is particularly vigilant about his blood flow and blood pressure. Cardio Miracle gives him greater confidence in strengthening himself against heart disease and regulating his blood pressure.

As Matsen measured his blood-pressure regularly, he discovered by his own data that after thirty days of supplementation with Cardio Miracle, his blood pressure was reduced from measurements as high as 170 all the way down to 118. Cardio Miracle has improved his health significantly. This was a testimony to him that Cardio Miracle isn't just a placebo, but that it actually works. Matsen also has gout, a disease which causes very painful swelling of certain smaller joints. He takes medication for gout, but he is monitoring his attacks of gout to see how better circulation helps him.

Matsen enjoys working out, but he doesn't like nitric oxide supplements that are packed with caffeine and other garbage. He takes a scoop of Cardio Miracle in water before his workouts because it is all natural, with no side-effects, and it produces better results than other nitric oxide supplements.

DOCTORS, PHYSICIANS, AND
OTHER MEDICAL PROFESSIONALS

Dr. Brad Nelson

For Dr. Bradley Nelson, author of The Emotion Code, Cardio Miracle is one of the few supplements that he and his wife take every single day. "The Cardio Miracle formula," Dr. Nelson asserts, "is superior to any formula" that he has ever used. He believes that everyone should take Cardio Miracle to protect and promote his or her health. In his own family there is a history of brain aneurysms. Dr. Nelson takes Cardio Miracle in the hope that it will minimize that risk for himself.

Dr. Joseph Prendergast

Doctor Prendergast helped to formulate and test several nitric oxide formulas for thousands of his patients over more than a decade. He was a committed Cardio Miracle user throughout the last decade. In his professional opinion, Cardio Miracle is "the finest nitric oxide product ever formulated in the marketplace."

Dr. Josh Helman

Blood pressure has been a major concern for Dr. Helman in his quest for excellent health. Nothing really seemed to help him until he discovered Cardio Miracle. Within three weeks of supplementing with Cardio Miracle twice a day, his blood pressure dropped to a normal range without medication. He was so grateful to find this amazing product.

Helman was skeptical when he first heard about Cardio Miracle, but the results for himself and his loved ones, along with his own research, confirmed that Cardio Miracle is the finest supplement that he has ever taken or evaluated. Helman believes that everyone should benefit from Cardio Miracle and prove the results for themselves as he has.

Dr. Christiane Northrup

When Dr. Northrup found out about Cardio Miracle, she knew that she had found an easy way for everyone to enjoy the health benefits of optimal nitric oxide levels. She has been recommending it ever since then, and she takes it herself. "This supplement," Northrup exclaimed, "is a game-changer!"

Jeff Hayes

"What people don't know," Jeff Hayes observed, "is that this product is driven by John's love for his fellow man. When Hayes saw how much time and money Hewlett was investing in Cardio Miracle, and what an outrageous risk he was taking, he recalls that Hewlett replied, "Jeff, people are dying, and I can stop this." From that point on, Hayes realized that there was no dissuading Hewlett or stopping him from accomplishing his mission.

Robert Scott Bell

Cardio Miracle has become an integral part of Robert Scott Bell's daily fitness routine as he pushes his body to higher levels of performance. Enhanced nitric oxide production has accelerated his recovery times as well. "If you want to operate at peak performance levels," Bell declared, "Cardio Miracle is a must!"

13

The Way Forward

I am honored to be considered one of America's Frontline Doctors (AFLDS) for such a time as this. To fight for medical and healthcare freedom and meaningful educational activities for so many. Thank you.

I am an African American with Native American heritage. I am proud to be in HIS family, from God's perspective

There are three groups of people in the world, based on God's perspective: the Jewish people, the Church, and the Gentiles (1Cor. 10:32).

I am a board-certified neurosurgeon, a vocation to which God called me at the age of 8 years old. 24 years later, I began to walk in that calling as a brain and spine surgeon.

I have performed thousands of surgeries since then. During medical school, internship, residency, and fellowship training, I was being indoctrinated in a very specific way of education. I thank the Lord, however, that He nudged me to question what I was hearing in recent years.

Pastor Mark Hankins introduced me to Dr Stella Emanuel in 2021, and my eyes were quickly opened.

Is Education Good or Bad?

Neither. Who controls the perspective from which education flows is key! Good or bad comes from the agenda of the entity that provides the information.

God's perspective is based on truth or the devils (worlds perspective) based on twisting parts of the truth.

Here is an Example of a medical education perspective:

Moyamoya disease is a rare, progressive cerebrovascular disorder caused by blocked arteries at the base of the brain in an area called the basal ganglia. Moyamoya means "puff of smoke" in Japanese. What gives this "puff of smoke" appearance on a CT scan, is the collection of tiny vessels that have formed over time to compensate for the blockage and find a way around it, in order to maintain adequate blood flow to the brain. This is known as neovascularization, and is God's creative miracle to our bodies, even in those fragile states.

What we see on a CT scan doesn't describe the **cause** of the problem. It doesn't describe the problem at all. It describes the radiologic appearance of our bodies' God-given **answer** to the problem.

It's an imaging finding of healing. It's not a disease at all. The vascular blockage is the problem. Yet in neurosurgery we call the natural, albeit incomplete, solution to the disease the disease itself. This is an example of an intellectual posture that the current medical education system (as part of the industrial biomedical complex) uses to call a symptom or a finding-the disease and that's what should be treated, primarily from a pharmaceutical/surgical standpoint, rather than the focus being on the root cause. A more common example is that of a fever. A fever in and of itself, is not a disease; it is a result or symptom of an underlying virus, bacteria, or other offender that our bodies' God-given answer to is to raise the body temperature to denature the proteins in the offender. Yet we use the term "treat" the fever, as though the fever itself is the root cause of ill health, when it is not. Should the body temperature be lowered when it is high enough to potentially cause organ damage? Of course! And me expounding on the use of slightly skewed terms like "treat a fever" and MoyaMoya "disease" may seem like such a minor detail, but it is "the little foxes that spoil the vines" (Song of Songs 2:15). If they can capture the words, no matter how skewed it is, it will affect that clinician's viewpoint of that thing.

You see: It's all about perspective and the motivation of medical education.

Education can be a stepping stone for advancement in every field but if it has no Governor of moral guidelines, then it becomes an exercise in futility whose relevance fades into an echo chamber of ideas and actions that seem productive, but takes on an empty path towards destruction.

The nation's first medical school opened in 1765 at the College of Philadelphia by John Morgan and William Shippen Jr.; this school developed over time into the University of Pennsylvania School of Medicine.

Medical schools created a classical system of continuing education; the first mandatory program was initiated in urology in 1934. By 1957, the first set of guidelines for medical practice were published by the American Medical Association (AMA).

Nathan Smith Davis Sr., M.D., LLD was a physician who established the American Medical Association in the 1860s and became the first editor of the Journal of the American Medical Association.

The mandatory nature of continuing education was widespread by the end of the 1960's. At the same time, the AMA created an honorary diploma for physicians.

Starting in 1970, the political predominance of the AMA in continuing education was questioned by other professional associations (hospitals, medical schools). After much discussion and opposing debate, a common association for continuing education was created in 1981. The AMA remained a leader in the early nineties and now has started programs targeted to patients.

In the middle of chaos God raised up the Association of American Physician and Surgeons (AAPS) in 1943 as a protector of independent doctors and the sanctity of the patient–physician relationship.

Continuing medical education consists of educational activities which serve to maintain, develop, or increase the knowledge, skills, and professional performance and relationships that a physician uses to provide services for patients, the public, or the profession.

Hosea 4:6 (KJV)

My people are destroyed for lack of knowledge: because thou hast rejected knowledge, I will also reject thee, that thou shalt be no priest to me: seeing thou hast forgotten the law of thy God, I will also forget thy children.

God speaks to our spirit (our heart- the real us)

We need to be educated in order to understand God's M. O. and who He is personally.

Science is one facet of God and a medium and process that He put in place to help us understand the natural phenomena that He created.

This is truth. He is truth.

Education void of a "God filter" and His precepts will never be as fruitful as it was meant to be. It will decay.

In 2016, After 15 years in neurosurgical practice, I was led to host and facilitate a knowledge sharing process in multiple fields of health and wellness connecting content experts who were top in their field from around the world. This program has continued since 2016.

We were led to add continuing medical education credits in order to allow participants of these sessions to receive recognized credit towards their maintenance of professional licensure in their specific areas of expertise from 2019.

In early 2021, a significant inflection point presented itself to me. I became even more aware of the lack of moral and scientific discipline, and the need to integrate the supernatural and natural by co-mingling social and intellectual learning with emphasis on wellness solutions of spirit, soul, and body.

We saw what was insane being called sane. We saw what was ethically **wrong** now being called ethically **right**.

My spiritual ministry, **The God Prescription** formed in 2018, and became a lightning rod to catalyze the origin of The Body Healthcare.

The Body Healthcare was formed in 2021 to **protect, organize, support, and educate** clinicians who pursue truth in care of their fellow humans.

We are at another inflection point in our great nation's history.

The ability to speak and apply truthful information in the care of people is threatened and has come under attack. Science has become **scientism**.

When it's acceptable to provide medical education credit for transgenderism that validates spiritual, emotional, and physical damage to our young people and yet deeply scientific presentations on life-saving low-risk, low-cost treatments are considered unscientific, then we have a real problem in our perception of scientific and academic rigor.

In 2021, Dr Stella Emanuel introduced me to Dr. Lee Vliet, former chair of the Association of American Physicians and Surgeons (AAPS). She told me that their amazing group of independent clinicians had their continuing medical education credits taken from them. Why?

Because they were advised in a letter that they were "biased" in their education programs because they presented information that was outside of the mandated protocols for treating COVID.

My company, now a subsidiary of The Body Healthcare, MNI Great Lakes-ECHO, partnered with AAPS (Association of American Physicians and Surgeons) to re-established their ability to provide these educational credits for support of professional licensure for their members at their educational events.

We were proud to support such an important entity in the history of medical practice and education. This is an example of what The Body Healthcare was created to do. We went on to support other organizations and their educational endeavors in a similar way.

In 2023, we sponsored a medical education conference for the Frontline Critical Care Consortium (FLCCC). They are a group of clinicians who were also very active in developing guidelines that were "outside the box" and helped to treat thousands of people during the COVID-19 pandemic. Just days before the conference began, an anonymous complaint was filed against our organization for sponsoring the conference of the FLCCC in order to receive continuing medical education credits. From the actual complaint: *the information to be communicated to attendees during this conference is misinformation and will not support any practicing physicians ability to better care for patients with COVID-19, it will only serve to make the care they provide uninformed and thus worse than if they had received no care at all.* We created a 2,000 page report in rebut of that complaint.

Ultimately, it didn't matter that there was overwhelming proof of scientific rigor in this conference that we provided medical education credit. The issue seemed to lie in a difference of opinion in treatment methodology. Our organization was placed on probation, along with the following request: *Regarding your 2022 activities, please provide Michigan State Medical Society a list of attendees for each activity including their names and state of residence.*

Remember Hosea 4:6

My people die for lack of knowledge because they rejected knowledge (of God's truth)...

We are more emboldened than ever to protect the health and well being of those we serve unencumbered by overreaching agencies that don't seem to validate the sanctity of the patient-physician relationship or the importance of unencumbered dissemination of medical education to better our ability to care for our patients.

We must create unique ways to educate ourselves and protect clinicians' ability to take care of members of society.

Our answer: **protect, organize. support, and educate** healthcare leaders, not political puppets of the biomedical industrial complex.

Out of chaos comes a virtual cornucopia of individuals determined to uphold the oath that they swore to God and those that they serve.

A private medical association like the AMA but with a twist. It answers to God only as its final authority.

It is literally a nonprofit church composed of principled men and women who care about the individual and have every intent to join forces with other independent groups that want to accomplish the same goals.

THE MISSION:
Protect

Organize

Support

Educate

- **Protect**–Dialog and open discussions as private membership in the exchange of knowledge and freedom to support wellness across the nation.

- **Organize**–Member-to-member networks to respond to dynamic opportunities across the nation.

- **Support** -Create communities for private advocacy. To support individual wellness clinics and those just starting up who are in need of support.

- **Educate**–Both clinicians and non-clinician members outside the current established systems with truth, validated data, and peer-reviewed journals that honor the Hippocratic Oath.

WE WILL NOT FALL ASLEEP ON THE JOB.

We are building alliances, connecting primary care practices from around the country. We are entering the educational curriculum phase as we begin creating primary functional wellness training programs and post graduate certification pathways to keep clinicians current. There will even be a medical publishing company to support and disseminate education and apply medical knowledge in a protected private membership model.

We are rebuilding trust within our clinical/ wellness communities around the country through hard work and a heart of love.

Please join our national private membership, promoting wellness in spirit, soul, and body at: www.thebodyhealthcare.com

References

Albesiano, Emilia, PhD, James E. Han, and Michael Lim, MD. "Mechanisms of Local Immunoresistance in Glioma." *Neurosurgery Clinics 21*, no. 1 (January 2010): 17–29.

American Psychological Association. "Stress in America: Our Health at Risk." January 11, 2012, https://www.apa.org/news/press/releases/ stress/2011/final-2011.pdf.

Antell, D. E., and E. M. Taczanowski. "How Environment and Lifestyle Choices Influence the Aging Process." *Annals of Plastic Surgery 43*, no. 6 (1999): 585–88.

Avena, N. M., P. Rada, and B. G. Hoebel. "Evidence for Sugar Addiction: Behavioral and Neurochemical Effects of Intermittent, Excessive Sugar Intake." *Neuroscience Biobehavior 32*, no. 1 (2008): 20–39.

Bain, G., D. Kitchens, M. Yao, et al. "Embryonic Stem Cells Express Neuronal Properties *in vitro*." *Developmental Biology 196* (1995): 342–57.

Barrès, Romain, et al. "Acute Exercise Remodels Promoter Methylation in Human Skeletal Muscle." *Cell Metabolism 15*, no. 3 (2012): 405.

Bendix, Jeffrey. "Opioid Policy Fallout." *Medical Economics*, June 10, 2018.

Benedict, Christian, et al. "Acute Sleep Deprivation Enhances the Brain's Response to Hedonic Food Stimuli: An fMRI Study." *The Journal of Clinical Endocrinology & Metabolism 97*, no. 3 (2012): E443–E447.

Buettner, Dan. *The Blue Zone: Lessons for Living Longer from the People Who've Lived the Longest.* Washington, DC: National Geographic, 2008. Kindle Edition.

Capps, Charles Emmitt. *God's Creative Power Will Work for You.* Tulsa, Oklahoma: Harrison House, 1976. (A minibook that organizes Scriptures into prayers)

Colcombe, Stanley J., et al. "Aerobic Exercise Training Increases Brain Volume in Aging Humans." *The Journals of Gerontology Series A: Biological Sciences and Medical Sciences 61*, no. 11 (2006): 1166–70.

Cotman, Carl W., and Nicole C. Berchtold. "Exercise: A Behavioral Intervention to Enhance Brain Health and Plasticity." *Trends in Neurosciences 25*, no. 6 (2002): 295–301.

Dempsey, Robert J., and Haviryaji S. G. Kalluri, PhD. "Ischemia- Induced Neurogenesis: Role of Growth Factors." *Neurosurgery Clinics of North America 18* (2007): 183–90.

Diamond, Adele, and Dima Amso. "Contributions of Neuroscience to Our Understanding of Cognitive Development. *Current Directions in Psychological Science 17*, no. 2 (2008): 136–41.

Fuerst, Mark L. "Underserved HCV Patients Benefiting from Telemedicine," *Medical Economics*, December 11, 2017, http://www.medicaleconomics.com/med-ec-blog/underserved-hcv- patients-benefiting-telemedicine.

Goldschlager, T., D. Oehme, P. Ghosh, et al. "Current and Future Applications for Stem Cell Therapies in Spine Surgery." *Current Stem Cell Research and Therapy Journal 8*, no. 5 (2013): 318–93.

Halberstadt, Craig, and Dwaine Emerich, eds. *Cellular Transplantation: From Laboratory to Clinic*. Amsterdam, the Netherlands: Elsevier, Inc. 2007.

Hassanzadeh, Hamid, MD, Isla Elboghdady, Junyoung Ahn, and Kern Singh, MD. "Basic Science of Mesenchymal Stem Cells in Spine Surgery." *Seminars in Spine Surgery 27* (2015): 72–75.

Hassanzadeh, Hamid, MD, and Kern Singh, MD, eds. "Mesenchymal Stem Cells in Spine Surgery." *Seminars in Spine Surgery 27* (2015): 72–75.

Hogue, David A. "Sensing the Other in Worship: Mirror Neurons and the Empathizing Brain." Liturgy 21, no. 3 (2006): 31–39.

Leaf, Caroline, PhD. *The Perfect You: A Blueprint for Identity*. Grand Rapids, Michigan: Baker Books, 2017.

Leaf, Caroline, PhD. *Think and Eat Yourself Smart: A Neuroscientific Approach to a Sharper Mind and Healthier Life*. Grand Rapids, Michigan: Baker Books, 2016.

Leaf, Caroline, PhD. *Who Switched Off My Brain? Controlling Toxic Thoughts and Emotions.* Nashville: Thomas Nelson Inc., 2009.

Lofgren, Ingrid Elizabeth. "Mindful Eating: An Emerging Approach for Healthy Manzel, Arndt, et al. "Role of 'Western Diet' in Inflammatory Autoimmune Diseases." *Current Allergy and Asthma Reports 14*, no. 1 (2014): 1–8.

McAfee, A. J., et al. "Red Meat from Animals Offered a Grass Diet Increases Plasma and Platelet N-3 PUFA in Healthy Consumers." *British Journal of Nutrition 105* (2011): 80–89.

Medical Economics. "Connect with Patients through Video." Josh Weiner. May 30, 2018, http://www.medicaleconomics.com/business/ connect-patients-through-video.

Medical Economics. "Opioid Abuse: Understand Guidelines to Protect Patients and Your Practice." Kelsey Boyle, Jon Heald, and Janis Coffin. May 30, 2018, http://www.medicaleconomics.com/business/opioid- abuse-understand-guidelines-protect-patients-and-your-practice.

Medical Economics. "What Patients Actually Want from Their Doctors." June 10, 2018, http://www.medicaleconomics.com/sites/default/files/ legacy/mm/digital/media/me061018_ezine.pdf.

Meyer, Joyce. *Battlefield of the Mind: Winning the Battle in Your Mind.* New York: Warner Books, Inc., 1995.

The Molecular Basis of Neurological Disease, vol. 8, a volume in Butterworths International Medical Reviews, Roger N. Rosenberg and A. E. Harding, eds. 1988.

Moore Life Ministries. "Careful for Nothing." Keith Moore. http://flcbranson.org/php/mlmMediaChannelCollectionContentList. php?site=mlm&channelID=1&languageID=EN&collectionID=173 &collectionName=Careful%20For%20Nothing.

Myckatyn, T. M., S. E. Mackinnon, and J. W. McDonald. "Stem Cell Transplantation and Other Novel Techniques for Promoting Recovery from Spinal Cord Injury." *Transplantation Immunology 12* (2004):343- 58.

Nader, Karim, Glenn E. Schafe, and Joseph E. Le Doux. "Fear Memories Require Protein Synthesis in the Amygdala for Reconsolidation After Retrieval." *Nature 406* (2000): 722–26.

The New York Times. "Rethinking Addiction's Roots and Its Treatment." Douglas Quenqua. July 10, 2011, http://www.nytimes. com/2011/07/11/health/11addictions.html.

Next Avenue.org. Friedman, Lawrence. "How the Mind-Gut Connection Affects Your Health. The 'Second Brain' in Your Stomach Can Cause or Relieve Illness and Stress. Here's How It Works." June 24, 2013, http://www.nextavenue.org/how-mind-gut-connection-affects- your-health/.

Newberg, Andrew, and Mark Robert Waldman. *How God Changes Your Brain: Breakthrough Findings from a Leading Neuroscientist.* New York: Ballantine, 2009.

Nikolai, Albert, PhD, and Trine Madsen, PhD. "Early Intervention Service for Young People with Psychosis: Saving Young Lives." *JAMA Psychiatry* (April 4, 2018).

Quiñones Hinojosa, Alfredo, MD, and Nader Sanai, MD. "Embryonic Human Stem Cells: Present and Future." *Neurosurgery Clinics of North America 18*, no. 1 (January 2007).

Richardson, R. Mark, MD, PhD, Dong Sun, MD, PhD, and M. Ross Bullock, MD, PhD. "Neurogenesis After Traumatic Brain Injury." *Neurosurgery Clinics of North America 18*, no. 1 (January 2007): 169-81.

Saavedra-Rodredra, Lorena, and Larry A. Feig. "Chronic Social Instability Induces Anxiety and Defective Social Interactions Across Generations. *Biological Psychiatry 73*, no. 1 (2013): 44–53.

Stiles, J. "Brain Development and the Nature Versus Nurture Debate." *Nature Genetics 33* (2003): 245–54.

Sugimura, Takashi, et al. "Heterocyclic Amines: Mutagens/ Carcinogens Produced During Cooking of Meat and Fish." *Cancer Science 95*, no. 4 (2004): 290–99.

TIME. "How Exercise Keeps Your DNA Young." Alice Park. July 27, 2016, http://time.com/4426572/ exercise-dna-telomeres/.

TIME. Special Edition. "The New Science of Exercise." Mandy Oaklander. September 12, 2016, http://time. com/4475628/the-new- science-of-exercise/.

TIME, Special Edition. "The Science of Exercise," Jordan D. Metzl, MD. 2017.

TIME, Special Edition. "The Science of Laughter: Our Bodies. Our Minds. Our Souls." June 28, 2018.

Seunggu, J. Han, Gurvinder Kaur, Isaac Yang, MD, and Michael Lim, MD. "Biologic Principles of Immunotherapy for Malignant Gliomas." *Neurosurgery Clinics of North America 21* (2010): 1–16.

Trepanowski, John F., and Richard J. Bloomer. "The Impact of Religious Fasting on Human Health." *Nutrition Journal 9* (2010): 57.

Waterland, R. A., and R. L. Jirtle. "Transposable Elements: Targets of Early Nutritional Effects on Epigenetic Gene Regulation." *Molecular Cell Biology 23*, no. 15 (2003): 5293–300.

Weinhold, Bob. "Epigenetics: The Science of Change." *Environmental Health Perspectives 114*, no. 3 (2006): A160–A167.

Whole Mind Project. "Whole Mind Shopping." March 8, 2017, http:// wholemindproject.com/whole-mind-living/whole-mind-shopping/.

Willett, W. C. "Balancing Lifestyle and Genomics Research for Disease Prevention." *Science 296* (2002): 695–98.

Wright, N. T. *Surprised by Scripture: Engaging Contemporary Issues.* San Francisco: HarperOne, 2014.

About the Author

Avery Jackson III, MD, FACS, FAANS Founder, CEO, and Medical Director Michigan Neurosurgical Institute, PC Grand Blanc, Michigan

Avery M. Jackson III, MD, is the chief executive officer and medical director of the Michigan Neurosurgical Institute, PC, which he founded in 2004. A board- certified neurosurgeon, Dr. Jackson has extensive training and experience in complex spinal cases, brain and spinal tumors, head and spine trauma, and minimally invasive procedures such as vertebroplasty and kyphoplasty to relieve pain. He is the proud founder of a fracture liaison service that helps manage and prevent osteoporosis and bone fractures due to osteoporosis and other bone diseases. He participates in several national registries.

Dr. Jackson participates in clinical trials of the latest neurosurgical treatments and techniques; frequently writes on medical audiences on neurosurgical topics; speaks to large audiences, both domestically and abroad; and holds several patents for medical inventions.

He held medical staff privileges at both Genesys Regional Medical Center and McLaren Regional Medical Center. He was the section head of the neurosurgery subsection at McLaren Regional Medical Center in Flint, Michigan, and served as the Chairman of Neurosurgery at Genesys Regional Medical Center in Grand Blanc, Michigan.

Previously, he served as attending staff neurosurgeon with Genesys Neurosurgical Associates. Prior to that, he was with Winchester Neurological Consultants in Winchester, Virginia. A graduate of the University of Chicago with a degree in biology, Dr. Jackson earned his medical degree at Wayne State University School of Medicine in Detroit and continued his training in general surgery at Northwestern University in Evanston, Illinois. He trained in neurosurgery at Penn State University, where he later served as Chief Resident in Neurosurgery at Milton S. Hershey Medical Center. Dr. Jackson also was a faculty instructor during a complex neurosurgical spine fellowship with the Medical College of Wisconsin.

Dr. Jackson served on numerous medical boards and was a member of several associations, including the American Medical Association, the American Association of Neurological Surgeons, the American College of Surgeons, the American Academy of Spine Physicians, the Michigan Association of Neurological Surgery, and the Michigan State Medical Society.

Dr. Jackson is the owner and founder of six companies:

1. Michigan Neurosurgical Institute, PC, neurosurgical practice, established 2004

2. MNI Great Lakes-ECHO LLC, an education and learning company, established 2016

3. Lindsay Marie Group, a land holding company, established in 2016

4. Optical Spine LLC, which owns surgical inventions, established in 2016

5. Freedom Innovations LLC, which owns surgical inventions, established in 2018

6. The Body Healthcare, A national private member to member 508c1a health and wellness business organization, established in 2021

The God Prescription
PO Box 210190
Auburn Hills, Michigan 48321

www.thegodprescription.com
www.thebodyhealthcare.com
Cardiomiracle.com/dravery

www.ingramcontent.com/pod-product-compliance
Lightning Source LLC
Chambersburg PA
CBHW061727270326
41928CB00011B/2140